INTERMITTENT FASTING FOR WOMEN OVER 50

JANICE ALEXANDER

COPYRIGHT

The information presented in this report solely and fully represents the views of the author as of the date of publication. Any omission, or potential Misrepresentation of, any peoples or companies, is entirely unintentional. As a result of changing information, conditions or contexts, this author reserves the right to alter content at their sole discretion impunity. The report is for informational purposes only and while every attempt has been made to verify the information contained herein, the author, assumes no responsibility for errors, inaccuracies, and omissions.Each person has unique needs and this book cannot take these individual differences in account.

Contents

INTRODUCTION

Intermittent Fasting (IF) refers to dietary eating patterns that involve not eating or severely restricting calories for a prolonged period of time. There are many different subgroups of intermittent fasting each with individual variation in the duration of the fast; some for hours, others for day(s). This has become an extremely popular topic in the science community due to all of the potential benefits on fitness and health that are being discovered.

Fasting, or periods of voluntary abstinence from food has been practiced throughout the world for ages. Intermittent fasting with the goal of improving health relatively new. Intermittent fasting involves restricting intake of food for a set period of time and does not include any changes to the actual foods you are eating. Currently, the most common IF protocols are a daily 16-hour fast and fasting for a whole day, one or two days per week. Intermittent fasting could be considered a natural eating pattern that humans are built to implement and it traces all the way back to our Paleolithic hunter-gatherer ancestors. The current model of a planned program of intermittent fasting could potentially help improve many aspects of health from body composition to longevity and aging. Although IF goes against the norms of our culture and common daily routine, the science may be pointing to less meal fre uency and more time fasting as the optimal alternative to the normal breakfast, lunch, and dinner model. Here are two common erroneous that pertain to intermittent fasting.

1 - You Must Eat 3 Meals Per Day: This "rule" that is common in Western society was not developed based on evidence for improved health, but was adopted as the common pattern for settlers and eventually became the norm. Not only is there a lack of scientific rationale in the 3 meal-a-day model, recent studies may

be showing less meals and more fasting to be optimal for human health. One study showed that one meal a day with the same amount of daily calories is better for weight loss and body composition than 3 meals per day. This finding is a basic concept that is extrapolated into intermittent fasting and those choosing to do IF may find it best to only eat 1-2 meals per day.

2 - You Need Breakfast, It's The Most Important Meal of the Day: Many false claims about the absolute need for a daily breakfast have been made. The most common claims being "breakfast increases your metabolism" and "breakfast decreases food intake later in the day". These claims have been refuted and studied over a 16-week period with results showing that skipping breakfast did not decrease metabolism and it did not increase food intake at lunch and dinner. It is still possible to do intermittent fasting protocols while still eating breakfast, but some people find it easier to eat a late

breakfast or skip it altogether and this common myth should not get in the way.

Intermittent fasting comes in various forms and each may have a specific set of unique benefits. Each form of intermittent fasting has variations in the fasting-to-eating ratio. The benefits and effectiveness of these different protocols may differ on an individual basis and it is important to determine which one is best for you. Factors that may influence which one to choose include health goals, daily schedule/routine, and current health status. The most common types of IF are alternate day fasting, time-restricted feeding, and modified fasting.

1. ALTERNATE DAY FASTING:

This approach involves alternating days of absolutely no calories (from food or beverage) with days of free feeding and eating whatever you want.

This plan has been shown to help with weight loss, improve blood cholesterol and triglyceride (fat) levels, and improve markers for inflammation in the blood.

The main downfall with this form of intermittent fasting is that it is the most difficult to stick with because of the reported hunger during fasting days.

2. MODIFIED FASTING - 5:2 DIET

Modified fasting is a protocol with programmed fasting days, but the fasting days do allow for some food intake. Generally, 20-25% of normal calories are allowed to be consumed on fasting days; so if you normally consume 2000 calories on regular eating days, you would be allowed 400-500 calories on fasting days. The 5:2 part of this diet refers to the ratio of non-fasting to fasting days. So on this regimen you would eat normally for 5 consecutive days, then fast or restrict calories to 20-25% for 2 consecutive days.

This protocol is great for weight loss, body composition, and may also benefit the regulation of blood sugar, lipids, and inflammation. Studies have shown the 5:2 protocol to be effective for weight loss, improve/lower inflammation markers in the blood (3), and show signs trending improvements in insulin resistance. In animal studies, this modified fasting 5:2 diet resulted in decreased fat, decreased hunger hormones (leptin), and increased levels of a protein responsible for improvements in fat burning and blood sugar regulation (adiponectin).

The modified 5:2 fasting protocol is easy to follow and has a small number of negative side effects which included hunger, low energy, and some irritability when beginning the program. Contrary to this however, studies have also noted improvements such as reduced tension, less anger, less fatigue, improvements in self-confidence, and a more positive mood.

3. TIME-RESTRICTED FEEDING:

If you know anyone that has said they are doing intermittent fasting, odds are it is in the form of time-restricted feeding. This is a type of intermittent fasting that is used daily and it involves only consuming calories during a small portion of the day and fasting for the remainder. Daily fasting intervals in time-restricted feeding may range from 12-20 hours, with the most common method being 16/8 (fasting for 16 hours, consuming calories for 8). For this protocol the time of day is not important as long as you are fasting for a consecutive period of time and only eating in your allowed time period. For example, on a 16/8 time-restricted feeding program one person may eat their first meal at 7AM and last meal at 3PM (fast from 3PM-7AM), while another person may eat their first meal at 1PM and last meal at 9PM (fast from

9PM-1PM). This protocol is meant to be performed every day over long periods of time and is very flexible as long as you are staying within the fasting/eating window(s).

Time-Restricted feeding is one of the easiest to follow methods of intermittent fasting. Using this along with your daily work and sleep schedule may help achieve optimal metabolic function. Time-restricted feeding is a great program to follow for weight loss and body composition improvements as well as some other overall health benefits. The few human trials that were conducted noted significant reductions in weight, reductions in fasting blood glucose, and improvements in cholesterol with no changes in perceived tension, depression, anger, fatigue, or confusion. Some other preliminary results from animal studies showed time restricted feeding to protect against obesity, high insulin levels, fatty liver disease, and inflammation.

The easy application and promising results of time-restricted feeding could possibly make it an excellent option for weight loss and chronic disease prevention/management. When implementing this protocol, it may be good to begin with a lower fasting-to-eating ratio like 12/12 hours and eventually work your way up to 16/8 hours.

While this book has been directed to women in their 50s, it is also a very useful resource for any gender of all age ranges.

THE SCIENCE BEHIND INTERMITTENT FASTING

While there is credible scientific evidence for intermittent fasting's benefits, it's neither a quick nor a guaranteed fix, according to leading researcher Satchin Panda. Panda, professor of circadian biology at the Salk Institute for Biological Studies in La Jolla, California, has spent his career studying the complex biochemical processes of the human body. His research — in mice and people — appears to suggest that intermittent fasting could benefit human health in a variety of different ways, including losing weight.

Before we dive into the science, let's put one thing up front: There's no one way to do intermittent fasting. If you google it, you'll find a menu of options, each with their own proponents. There's the 5: 2 diet, which involves eating very few calories (roughly 500-600) for two days of the week, followed by five days of normal eating. Or, there's alternate-day fasting, which means eating normally one day and then eating either nothing or just 500 calories the next.

All intermittent fasting methods are essentially based on the same idea: When you reduce your caloric intake, your body will use its stored fat for energy. But what makes intermittent fasting different from simply cutting calories is the possibility that it's easier for people to restrict calories for limited stretches of time rather than for the days, weeks and months demanded by conventional diets. Plus, the specific type of intermittent fasting that Panda has studied may have additional positive effects.

Panda has focused on an intermittent fasting method known as time-restricted eating. In this format, a person consumes all of their calories for the day within an 8-to-12-hour window. Let's say you usually start your day with a first cup of coffee at 7AM and eventually wind down with popcorn and a drink around 11PM. With time-restricted eating, you might switch to eating breakfast at 8AM, including coffee, and finishing your dinner by 6PM. That way, you're eating all your meals within a 10-hour window — and you're most likely forgoing calories from desserts, evening snacks and alcohol. But that's not the whole story.

Time-restricted eating seems to be doing more for the body than simply reducing calorie intake. This was first suggested by a 2012 study that Panda and colleagues did with mice. They took two genetically identical sets of mice and fed them the same diet — a lab-mice version of the standard American diet that's high in fat and simple sugar and low in protein.

While both groups were given the exact same amount of food, one group had access to the food for 24 hours and the other group had access to it for only 8 hours. Mice are nocturnal, typically sleeping during the day and eating at night. But when one group was given round-the-clock access to food, those mice began eating some of it during the day as well, when they'd normally be sleeping.

After 18 weeks, the mice who could eat at all hours showed signs of insulin resistance and also had liver damage. But the mice who ate in an 8-hour window did not have these conditions. They also weighed 28 percent less than the mice with 24-hour access to food — even though both groups of mice ate the same number of calories a day. "It was kind of earth-shattering," Panda recalls. Until then, he says that he and other researchers had thought the total number of calories, rather than when they were eaten, were what determined weight gain.

His team repeated the experiment with three additional sets of mice and got the same results. The outcomes also held steady for different types of food and for eating windows of up to 15 hours — although, interestingly, the shorter the window, the less weight the mice gained. When the time-restricted mice were switched over to unrestricted eating for two days a week, or what Panda calls "having the weekend off", they still gained less weight than the mice allowed to eat 24 hours a day.

Then, Panda's team also tried it another way: They took mice that had gained weight because of unrestricted feeding and switched them to time-restricted eating. Despite eating the same amount of calories, these mice lost weight and maintained it for 12 weeks until the end of the study. They also reduced their insulin resistance, which is thought to be linked to obesity, although scientists still don't understand the association. Of course, the human body is more complex than that of a mouse, Panda says, but these experiments were the first indication of how important timing could be when it comes to how our bodies use food.

In recent years, scientists have been discovering that so many of the human body's processes are tied to our circadian rhythms. For example, most of us know that getting sunlight early in the morning is beneficial to our mood and sleep and that being exposed to light at 9PM via our cell phones or laptops can disrupt our night's sleep. "Similarly, food at the right time can nurture us, and healthy food at the wrong time can be junk food," Panda says. Instead of being used as fuel, it gets stored as fat, which makes sense once you examine the basics of how human metabolism works.

Time-restricted eating gives our body more time to use up fat. When we eat, our body uses carbohydrates for energy, and if we don't need them right away, they get stored in the liver as glycogen or converted into fat. After we've finished eating for the day, our body continues to run on glucose from the carbohydrates that we've just eaten for a few hours before tapping into stored carbohydrates, or glycogen, in the liver. That glycogen lasts for several hours before running out roughly eight hours after we've stopped eating, which is when our body begins to tap into its stored fat.

When we shorten our eating window and extend our fasting window, we spend longer in this fat-burning mode of our metabolism. But the moment we ingest food again — even if it's just coffee with a bit of sugar and milk — we switch back into the other mode and start burning carbohydrates and storing glycogen and fat. So if you finish eating at 10PM with your evening snack, your body will run out of glycogen and start burning fat at around 6AM. If you usually eat breakfast at 6AM but you change that to 9AM, you've given your body three extra hours to use fat as fuel.

Panda followed up his time-restricted eating experiments in humans — and found it showed promise there, too. In 2015, he and his colleagues tried putting small group of people on a time-restricted eating plan for 16 weeks. Intriguingly, the researchers gave these people no diet instructions or advice at all. Instead, the subjects were told to choose a 10-to-12 hour window in which to do all their eating. When they ate, they took pictures of their food and texted it to the researchers. After 16 weeks, the subjects showed a small amount of weight loss — an average of just over 8 pounds each. But they reported experiencing better sleep, more energy in the mornings and less hunger at bedtime, suggesting time-restricted eating "actually has a systemic impact all over the body," according to Panda. While it was much too small a group of people to be able to draw definitive conclusions, the researchers found it encouraging that this simple intervention seemed easy for subjects to implement and sustain.

Time-restricted eating has shown some potential to prevent diabetes. In a study of 15 men at risk for type-2 diabetes that was run by Panda, he and his team found that after one week of limiting them to eating within a nine-hour window, the men showed a lower spike in blood glucose after a test meal, a sign of improved insulin sensitivity. It might also help lower cholesterol. In another experiment, Panda and colleagues had 19 people — most of whom were on medication to lower cholesterol or blood pressure or treat diabetes — time-restrict their eating. After 12 weeks of eating within a 10-hour window, they lowered their total cholesterol by about 11 percent on average. What's more, Panda checked in one year later and found that roughly ¾ of the subjects were still voluntarily eating in an 8-11 hour window. "It was gratifying that they could self-sustain this for a period of time," Panda says. This is good news given that by some estimates, ⅓ to ½ of dieters eventually regain more weight than they lose.

Here's how you can practice time-restricted eating, according to Panda. While some intermittent fasting plans allow people to have unlimited quantities of coffee and tea during the day, he says you should consume only water during your fasting window. This means no coffee, tea or herbal tea, which can all change blood chemistry and which is why they're not allowed during fasts for medical blood tests.

Panda recommends that you drink plain hot water after you wake up; it can give you some of the same soothing feeling as coffee. Of course, if it's important for you to be alert in the morning, he says it's OK to have some black coffee — but stay away from any adding creamer, sugar, honey or other sweeteners. "Just one teaspoon of sugar is enough to double our blood sugar," he says, and switches your body out of fat-burning mode and back into carb-burning mode.

As to when to have your meals, Panda recommends that you wait to eat breakfast until you've been awake for a couple of hours. About 45 minutes after you wake up, the hormone cortisol spikes and high cortisol levels can impede your glucose regulation. Plus, the hormone melatonin, which prepares our body for sleep, only wears off about two hours after waking. This means that, for those first two hours, your pancreas, which produces the insulin needed to use carbohydrates in food, is also just waking up. Then you should try to finish your last meal about two to three hours before your bedtime since that's when the melatonin begins to prepare the body, including your pancreas, for sleep.

While intermittent fasting, and time-restricted eating in particular, holds tantalizing promise, it's still early days. Since Panda began his research, other research groups have backed up some of his results. For example, a study published in July in Cell Metabolism found that people on a time-restricted eating program reduced their calorie intake, even though they weren't asked to, and lost a modest amount of weight.

There's a need for more research about time-restricted eating. So far, there haven't been any studies with human subjects that lasted longer than a few months. Researchers also need to understand the ways in which fasting affects the human body. For example, the gut microbiome has been shown to actually change in mice that restrict their eating to an eight-nine hour window so that they digest nutrients differently, absorbing less sugar and fat. Is this possible in humans? That remains to be seen. Panda is not the only one investigating the effects of time-restricted eating that go beyond weight loss; other researchers are also beginning to explore whether intermittent fasting might also protect the brain from neurodegenerative diseases.

Intermittent fasting is not a silver bullet for weight loss. Some research even suggests that people practicing the 5:2 diet or alternate-day fasting might instinctively eat more before and after their fasting days or reduce their activity on fasting days, negating the calorie-reducing benefits. In his studies of time-restricted eating, Panda says he's seen some participants gain weight after they've taken the idea of eating whatever they wanted within a window to the extreme, bingeing on the foods they usually abstained from. Also, unlike mice, the human body may have ways of slowing down metabolism so that as you consume fewer calories, you also burn fewer. Finally, it's unclear whether intermittent fasting is beneficial for people who aren't trying to lose weight. In fact, there's a potential danger for people who struggle with binge-eating disorder or anorexia; it's not hard to see how attempting intermittent fasting could encourage these harmful behaviors.

Time-restricted eating has practical advantages over other dieting options: It's easy and accessible. Many people don't have the time or resources to count calories — planning their meals, buying certain foods, tracking their calories — so that diets are often the privilege of people who can afford them. Time-restricted eating can be done by anyone who can count time and limit eating and drinking to specific periods.

Panda and his colleagues are now conducting a study of time-restricted eating to 120 participants. They're also investigating whether firefighters might improve their health by eating in a 10-hour window. Firefighters and other shift workers are more prone to disease due to the constant disruption to their circadian rhythms.

For a long time, people who want to lose weight have had to focus on changing the foods on their daily menus. Time-restricted eating has the potential of expanding the factors that we could control. "When it comes to health, we have a menu" of options, says Panda, who adheres to a 10-hour window of eating. "Now we can add the timing of food to the menu.

There are some interesting updates on the concept of Intermittent Fasting and how it works.

There's a ton of incredibly promising intermittent fasting (IF) research done on fat rats. They lose weight, their blood pressure, cholesterol, and blood sugars improve… but they're rats. Studies in humans, almost across the board, have shown that IF is safe and incredibly effective, but really no more effective than any other diet. In addition, many people find it difficult to fast.

But a growing body of research suggests that the timing of the fast is key, and can make IF a more realistic, sustainable, and effective approach for weight loss, as well as for diabetes prevention.

It makes intuitive sense that Intermittent fasting can help weight loss. The food we eat is broken down by enzymes in our gut and eventually ends up as molecules in our bloodstream. Carbohydrates, particularly sugars and refined grains (think white flours and rice), are quickly broken down into sugar, which our cells use for energy. If our cells don't use it all, we store it in our fat cells as, well, fat. But sugar can only enter our cells with insulin, a hormone made in the pancreas. Insulin brings sugar into the fat cells and keeps it there.

Between meals, as long as we don't snack, our insulin levels will go down and our fat cells can then release their stored sugar, to be used as energy. We lose weight if we let our insulin levels go down. The entire idea of IF is to allow the insulin levels to go down far enough and for long enough that we burn off our fat.

Intermittent fasting can be hard… but maybe it doesn't have to be

Initial human studies that compared fasting every other day to eating less every day showed that both worked about equally for weight loss, though people struggled with the fasting days. So, I had written off IF as no better or worse than simply eating less, only far more uncomfortable. My advice was to just stick with the sensible, plant-based, Mediterranean-style diet.

New research is suggesting that not all IF approaches are the same, and some are actually very reasonable, effective, and sustainable, especially when combined with a nutritious plant-based diet. So I'm prepared to take my lumps on this one.

We have evolved to be in sync with the day/night cycle, i.e., a circadian rhythm. Our metabolism has adapted to daytime food, nighttime sleep. Nighttime eating is well associated with a higher risk of obesity, as well as diabetes.

Based on this, researchers from the University of Alabama conducted a study with a small group of obese men with prediabetes. They compared a form of intermittent fasting called "early time-restricted feeding," where all meals were fit into an early eight-hour period of the day (7 am to 3 pm),or spread out over 12 hours (between 7 am and 7 pm). Both groups maintained their weight (did not gain or lose) but after five weeks, the eight-hours group had dramatically lower insulin levels and significantly improved insulin sensitivity, as well as significantly lower blood pressure. The best part? The eight-hours group also had significantly decreased appetite. They weren't starving.

Just changing the timing of meals, by eating earlier in the day and extending the overnight fast, significantly benefited metabolism even in people who didn't lose a single pound.

Why might changing timing help?

But why does simply changing the timing of our meals to allow for fasting make a difference in our body? An in-depth review of the science of IF recently published in New England Journal of Medicine sheds some light. Fasting is evolutionarily embedded within our physiology, triggering several essential cellular functions. Flipping the switch from a fed to fasting state does more than help us burn calories and lose weight. The researchers combed through dozens of animal and human studies to explain how simple fasting improves metabolism, lowering blood sugar; lessens inflammation, which improves a range of health issues from arthritic pain to asthma; and even helps clear out toxins and damaged cells, which lowers risk for cancer and enhances brain function.

So, is intermittent fasting as good as it sounds?

So, here's the deal. There is some good scientific evidence suggesting that circadian rhythm fasting, when combined with a healthy diet and lifestyle, can be a particularly effective approach to weight loss, especially for people at risk for diabetes. (However, people with advanced diabetes or who are on medications for diabetes, people with a history of eating disorders like anorexia and bulimia, and pregnant or breastfeeding women should not attempt intermittent fasting unless under the close supervision of a physician who can monitor them.)

INTERMITTENT FASTING AND GENDER

Although gender can be a sensitive and controversial subject, differences between men and women are important to consider in relationship to health. Political, economic, and cultural arguments aside, biology has formulated men and women differently at a genetic (and thus phenotypic) level. The differences between men and women go beyond X and Y chromosomes. We can see these differences in the fact that men are on average taller than women and the fact that women generally have smaller lungs.

How Does Intermittent Fasting Impact Women vs. Men?

Gender roles dictated by biology have played a part in shaping male and female metabolic responses to exercise, carbohydrates, sleep deprivation, and yes — you guessed it — fasting.

While living in hunter-gatherer societies, men and women adapted to periods of plenty and scarcity differently. Men, with their generally larger physical size, responded to fasting with a giant boost in metabolic rate. This metabolic boost gave them the fuel necessary to hunt. Essentially, men's genetic makeup says, "Go get food for everyone," when they haven't had much to eat.

Research reveals that genetic adaptations to periods of scarcity can still be seen in humans today. During short periods of fasting (twelve to twenty-four hours) men's metabolisms increase up to 14 percent. Other effects of intermittent fasting on the male body include an increase between 10 and 200 percent in testosterone utilization, an increase between 100 and 200 percent in growth hormone, and an improvement in blood lipids to support the increased hormonal production and decreased risk factors for cardiovascular disease.

Women, however, do not respond to intermittent fasting like men do. In hunter-gatherer societies, women's bodies responded to periods of scarcity differently than the bodies of men did. Women's metabolisms slowed down to conserve energy and store fat in order to survive a potential long-term famine. What this means for women today is that intermitting fasting may not work well for their bodies.

Do Hormones Impact How Intermittent Fasting Works?

Some hormones, which we can call "hunger hormones," have an impact on how hungry we feel. And these hunger hormones impact how intermittent fasting works. The two important hunger hormones are leptin and ghrelin. Created by fat cells, leptin decreases your appetite or level of hunger. Ghrelin, in contrast, is an appetite stimulator. The stomach releases ghrelin, which is believed to signal hunger to the brain.

Research suggests that intermittent fasting can lower levels of ghrelin. This, in turn, can lead to lower feelings of hunger and weight loss.

Is There Any Research Being Done on How Intermittent Fasting Impacts Men and Women?

Research on intermittent fasting demonstrates gender ineuality. Out of seventy-one studies found in Harvard's database for intermittent fasting, only thirteen include women at all. Beyond that, absolutely none of the controlled studies focus on the female population in general. There are no controlled studies that allow us to draw intelligent conclusions about how intermittent fasting affects the female population.

One of the thirteen studies related to intermittent fasting that includes women is on pregnant women fasting during Ramadan. This study found no improvement in insulin sensitivity and an increase in blood lipids for women. This suggests that at least some of the health benefits touted by other studies of intermittent fasting apply only to men. Additionally, as every woman who has been pregnant knows, the female body is completely different when pregnant versus not pregnant.

When you sift through the precious little data on women in a fasted state, you find something fascinating: women don't respond to fasting like men do.

In fact, instead of much-celebrated metabolic boosts and weight loss, women might find a 50 percent increase in cortisol and a decrease in insulin sensitivity as a result of intermittent fasting. This means that intermittent fasting could contribute to obesity and diabetes instead of health benefits for women.

Which Gender Does Better with Intermittent Fasting?

Overall, men tend to do better with intermittent fasting. They experience the most proven health benefits from this style of eating. Women, in contrast, tend to benefit from other diets and eating styles discussed below.

Intermittent Fasting and Women

Although we could benefit from more research on this subject, women should consider what we do know about intermittent fasting before deciding to try this eating style.

ISSA, International Sports Sciences Association, Certified Personal Trainer, ISSAonline, Intermittent Fasting: Women vs. Men

Is Intermittent Fasting a Good Weight-Loss Diet for Women?

As suggested above, an intermittent fasting diet is likely not going to help women lose weight. Men are likely to benefit from skipping breakfast or restricting their calorie intake for an entire day once or twice a week. These actions can boost metabolism and lead to weight loss. Women, however, are not likely to benefit from the same diet.

Women who want to optimize their body composition, have consistently high energy, and continually improve their workout performance would benefit the most from a constant calorie intake each day. An unchanging flow of high-quality calories — rather than intermittent fasting — is likely to lead to the best weight loss results for women.

Do Women Get Enough Nutrients on Intermittent Fasting Diets?

Intermittent fasting might actually prevent women from getting enough nutrients. By maintaining an unchanging flow of high-quality calories, women can ensure that they are getting enough nutrients to maximize their health. Because of this, women, more than men, might benefit from sticking to the old guideline of eating four to six small meals per day.

WHAT KIND OF WOMEN SHOULD AND SHOULDN'T TRY INTERMITTENT FASTING?

Women who are trying to become pregnant should not try intermittent fasting. Diets with consistent food intake rather than severe calorie restrictions are particularly important for women who want to conceive. This is because intermittent fasting can impact a woman's menstrual cycle, leading to missed periods and infertility.

Intermittent fasting does not only have to be for men. However, we recommend that women ask their doctors about fasting and consider the potential health benefits and risks before trying this or any diet.

THE SCIENCE BEHIND INTERMITTENT FASTING

Something that is particularly fascinating for trainers is the impact of limited research on health and fitness recommendations and practices.

Why are there so many different recommendations out there? Why do some experts recommend a high-carb diet while others recommend a low-carb diet for maximum health? Or weight training versus cardio training for fat loss? Or volume versus intensity for exercise? The answer can often be found in the way that scientific research is conducted. Focused research on one type of individual is likely to produce different results than focused research on a different type of individual.

Research on the science of intermittent fasting—especially for women—still has a long way to go. That said, individuals who are interested in trying this type of diet can be confident that there is some science behind intermittent fasting.

What Body Chemicals Are Impacted by Intermittent Fasting?

Intermittent fasting affects many chemicals in the body, including the hunger hormones leptin and ghrelin. As discussed above, intermittent fasting reduces ghrelin and can help you lose weight.

In addition to helping with weight loss, intermittent fasting can lead to lower blood sugar and insulin levels, lower LDL ("bad") cholesterol and blood triglycerides, and reduced inflammation. It is important to note, however, that most research on how intermittent fasting affects body chemicals comes from studies done on men.

Is There Any Science Behind Intermittent Fasting?

There is certainly science behind the intermittent fasting diet. That said, it is good advice to be skeptical of any newly hyped diet or exercise fad that claims to be effective for everyone. One size does not fit all. This is a core reason why our industry exists.

Inherently, we know men and women need different things from us as trainers, in the same way that people of different ages, training experience levels, and body types need different things from us as trainers. We hope that the science of nutrition and exercise will catch up to our intuition as trainers one day.

TYPES OF INTERMITTENT FASTING

5:2 Fasting

5:2 intermittent fasting works by allotting five days a week to practice normal eating habits and two days of reduced caloric intake. Meaning during these two days no more than 500 calories should be consumed. These two days of fasting do not necessarily come right after the five non-fasting days. They can be intermixed throughout the week.

The 5:2 diet plan has proven to be a successful tool for combating weight gain, and decreasing insulin resistance.

16/8 Daily Fasting

The 16/8 intermittent daily fasting routine allows you to eat for eight hours followed by a fasting period of 16 hours. This fasting period includes sleep time, so there is no need to worry about sleep negatively affecting the fast.

To increase the efficiency of IF, experts advise to fit in at least two or three small meals throughout the eating window. Many people have vouched for daily fasting as being the easiest way that burns calories fast, even in women of older ages.

Eat Stop Eat

Eat stop eat, also known as alternate-day fasting, includes a 'feeding day,' where the person can eat whatever they want (within moderation and still eating healthy) for one whole day, followed with a 'fasting day,' where the normal caloric intake is reduced to 25% for the next 24 hours. On the fasting day, it is advised to eat more protein, vegetables, and healthy fats and reduce the intake of sugar or starches.

Eat stop eat method can be done from breakfast to breakfast or from lunch to lunch. This type of intermittent fast can prove to be a bit tricky and is, therefore, suitable for advanced fasters.

BENEFITS OF INTERMITTENT FASTING FOR WOMEN OVER 50

A few things that make it tougher to lose weight after age 50 include lower metabolism, achy joints, reduced muscle mass, and even sleep issues. At the same time, losing fat, especially dangerous belly fat, can dramatically reduce your risk for such serious health issues as diabetes, heart attacks, and cancer.

Of course, as you age, the risk of developing many diseases increases. In some cases, intermittent fasting for women over 50 could serve as a virtual fountain of youth when it comes to weight loss and minimizing the chance of developing typically age-related illnesses.

HOW DOES INTERMITTENT FASTING WORK?

Intermittent fasting, often referred to as IF, won't force you to starve yourself. It also doesn't give you a license to consume lots of unhealthy food during the time when you don't fast. Instead of eating meals and snacks all day, you eat within a specific window of time.

Most people make an IF schedule that re◻uires them to fast for 12 to 16 hours a day. During the rest of the time, they eat normal meals and snacks. Sticking to this eating window isn't as hard as it sounds because most people sleep for about eight of their fasting hours. In addition, you're encouraged to enjoy zero-calorie drinks, like water, tea, and coffee.

You should develop an eating schedule that works for you for the best intermittent fasting results. For instance:

• 12-hour fasts: With a 12-12 fast, you might simply skip breakfast and wait to eat until lunch. If you prefer to eat your morning meal, you could eat an early supper and avoid evening snacks. Most older women find a 12-12 fast pretty easy to stick to.

• 16-hour fasts: You may enjoy faster results with a 16-8 IF schedule. Most people choose to consume two meals and a snack or 2 a day within an 8-hour window. For example, you might set your eating window between noon and 8 in the evening or between 8 in the morning and 4 in the afternoon.

• 5-2 schedule: Restricted eating periods may not work for you every day. Another alternative is to stick to a 12- or 16-hour fast for 5 days and then relax your schedule for 2 days. For instance, you might use IF during the week and eat normally on the weekend.

• Every-other-day fasts: Another variation calls for very restricted calories on alternate days. For example, you might keep your calories under 500 on one day and then eat normally the next day. Note that daily IF fasts never call for restricting calories that low.

As with any diet, you'll get the best results if you're consistent. At the same time, you can certainly give yourself a break from this kind of eating schedule on special occasions. You should experiment to figure out which kind of intermittent fasting works the best for you. Lots of people ease themselves into IF with the 12-12 plan, and then they progress to 16-8. After that, you should try to stick to that plan as much as possible.

Some people believe that IF has worked for them simply because the limited eating window naturally helps them reduce the number of calories they consume. For instance, instead of eating 3 meals and 2 snacks, they might find that they only have time for 2 meals and one snack. They become more mindful about the kinds of food they consume and tend to stay away from processed carbs, unhealthy fat, and empty calories.

Of course, you can also choose the kinds of healthy food that you enjoy. While some people opt to reduce their overall calorie intake, others combine IF with a keto, vegan, or other kinds of diets.

BEYOND CALORIE RESTRICTION

While some nutrition experts contend that IF only works because it helps people naturally limit food intake, others disagree. They believe that intermittent fasting results are better than typical meal schedules with the same amount of calories and other nutrients. Studies have even suggested that abstaining from food for several hours a day does more than just limit the number of calories you consume.

These are some metabolic changes that IF causes that might help account for synergistic benefits:

• Insulin: During the fasting period, lower insulin levels will help improve fat burning.

• HGH: While insulin levels drop, HGH levels rise to encourage fat burning and muscle growth.

• Noradrenaline: In response to an empty belly, the nervous system will send this chemical to cells to let them know they need to release fat for fuel.

HOW SAFE?

Is intermittent fasting safe? Remember that you're only supposed to fast for 12 to 16 hours and not for days at a time. You've still got plenty of time to enjoy a satisfying and healthy diet. Of course, some older women may need to eat fre🞏uently because of metabolic disorders or instructions on prescriptions. In that case, you should discuss your eating habits with your medical provider before making any changes.

While it's not technically fasting, some doctors have reported intermittent fasting benefits by allowing such easy-to-digest food as whole fruit during the fasting window. Modifications like these can still give your digestive and metabolic system a needed rest.

In fact, the authors of the work said that they had patients who only changed their eating habits with this 12- to 16-hour "fruit" fast each day. They did not follow the diet's other rules or count calories, and they still lost weight and got healthier. This strategy might have simply worked because the dieters replaced junk food with whole foods. In any case, people found this dietary change effective and easy to make. Traditionalists won't call this fasting; however, it's important to know that you may have options if you absolutely can't abstain from food for several hours at a time.

Dr. Becky, a chiropractor and over-50 fitness consultant, says it's tough to find any downsides to IF in the medical literature. She explained that during the fasting period, your blood sugar and insulin levels will drop to low levels. Without insulin's hormonal fat-storing signal, your body will rely upon stored fat for energy.

IS INTERMITTENT FASTING THE BEST FAT-LOSS TOOL FOR YOU?

In any case, IF appears to work mostly because people find it fairly easy to adhere to. They say it helps them naturally limit calories and make better food choices by reducing eating windows. Some studies suggest that IF is better than only cutting calories, carbs, or fat because it appears to promote fat loss while sparing lean muscle mass.

Of course, most people use IF with another weight-loss plan. For instance, you might decide to eat 1,200 calories a day to lose weight. You may find it much easier to spread out 1,200 calories within 2 meals and 2 snacks than in 3 meals and 3 snacks. If you've struggled with weight loss because your diet either didn't work or was simply too hard to stick to, you might try intermittent fasting for quicker results.

GENERAL BENEFITS

Being one of the hottest topics in the weight loss world, intermittent fasting has proven itself as a successful remedy for losing weight, maintaining muscle mass, increasing longevity, and even enhancing cognition. Above all, it is considered to be widely useful for older women who want to lose belly fat.

- Reduces Weight: Belly fat becomes an issue for women as soon as they hit the age 40, not only due to its bad appearance but also because of its deteriorating effects on the general health. Weight loss through intermittent fasting enables such post-menopausal women to reduce their risk of encountering several life-threatening diseases.

- Strengthens Musculoskeletal System: Intermittent fasting for women over 50 has been clinically proven to enhance the overall health of the skeletal system. It has been found to be an efficient way of reducing the symptoms of arthritis and back pain which are commonly encountered by older women. A few studies have also proven how altering meal plans according to IF can affect the production of hormones that control muscle and bone health. Research has proven that fasting helps to reduce pathways that increase the production of cancerous cells. Intermittent fasting for women over 50 can aid an increase in self-esteem and better moods along with a decrease in negative symptoms like anxiety, depression, and stress.

- Controls Diabetes: Eating during certain periods of time is strongly correlated with a decreased risk of diabetes. Some studies show that intermittent fasting can be an efficient way to keep glucose levels in check, get off insulin, and even get rid of, or reduce the usage of prescribe medications.

- Improves Longevity : When a women starts fasting at fixed intervals, their body starts sending a signal that activates genetic repair mechanism. This mechanism fights aging and various other diseases by producing human growth hormone (HGH). HGH, in turn, works to strengthen muscles, ligaments, and tendons, speed up metabolic rate, regenerate tissues and increase longevity. This is arguably one of the best advantages of intermittent fasting for women over 50.

WEIGHT LOSS & DIABETES

First of all, fasting is not starvation. Starvation is the involuntary abstinence from eating forced upon by outside forces; this happens in times of war and famine when food is scarce. Fasting, on the other hand, is voluntary, deliberate, and controlled. Food is readily available but we choose not to eat it due to spiritual, health, or other reasons.

Fasting is as old as mankind, far older than any other forms of diets. Ancient civilizations, like the Greeks, recognized that there was something intrinsically beneficial to periodic fasting. They were often called times of healing, cleansing, purification, or detoxification. Virtually every culture and religion on earth practice some rituals of fasting.

Before the advent of agriculture, humans never ate three meals a day plus snacking in between. We ate only when we found food which could be hours or days apart. Hence, from an evolution standpoint, eating three meals a day is not a requirement for survival. Otherwise, we would not have survived as a species.

Fast forward to the 21st century, we have all forgotten about this ancient practice. After all, fasting is really bad for business! Food manufacturers encourage us to eat multiple meals and snacks a day. Nutritional authorities warn that skipping a single meal will have dire health consequences.

Overtime, these messages have been so well-drilled into our heads.

Fasting has no standard duration. It may be done for a few hours to many days to months on end. Intermittent fasting is an eating pattern where we cycle between fasting and regular eating. Shorter fasts of 16-20 hours are generally done more fre?uently, even daily. Longer fasts, typically 24-36 hours, are done 2-3 times per week. As it happens, we all fast daily for a period of 12 hours or so between dinner and breakfast.

Fasting has been done by millions and millions of people for thousands of years. Is it unhealthy? No. In fact, numerous studies have shown that it has enormous health benefits.

What Happens When We Eat Constantly?

Before going into the benefits of intermittent fasting, it is best to understand why eating 5-6 meals a day or every few hours (the exact opposite of fasting) may actually do more harm than good.

When we eat, we ingest food energy. The key hormone involved is insulin (produced by the pancreas), which rises during meals. Both carbohydrates and protein stimulate insulin. Fat triggers a smaller insulin effect, but fat is rarely eaten alone.

Insulin has two major functions -

First, it allows the body to immediately start using food energy. Carbohydrates are rapidly converted into glucose, raising blood sugar levels. Insulin directs glucose into the body cells to be used as energy. Proteins are broken down into amino acids and excess amino acids may be turned into glucose.

Protein does not necessarily raise blood glucose but it can stimulate insulin. Fats have minimal effect on insulin.

Second, insulin stores away excess energy for future use. Insulin converts excess glucose into glycogen and store it in the liver. However, there is a limit to how much glycogen can be stored away. Once the limit is reached, the liver starts turning glucose into fat. The fat is then put away in the liver (in excess, it becomes fatty liver) or fat deposits in the body (often stored as visceral or belly fat).

Therefore, when we eat and snack throughout the day, we are constantly in a fed state and insulin levels remain high. In other words, we may be spending the majority of the day storing away food energy.

What Happens When We Fast?

The process of using and storing food energy that occurs when we eat goes in reverse when we fast. Insulin levels drop, prompting the body to start burning stored energy. Glycogen, the glucose that is stored in the liver, is first accessed and used. After that, the body starts to break down stored body fat for energy.

Thus, the body basically exists in two states - the fed state with high insulin and the fasting state with low insulin. We are either storing food energy or we are burning food energy. If eating and fasting are balanced, then there is no weight gain. If we spend the majority of the day eating and storing energy, there is a good chance that overtime we may end up gaining weight.

Intermittent Fasting Versus Continuous Calorie-Restriction

The portion-control strategy of constant caloric reduction is the most common dietary recommendation for weight loss and type 2 diabetes. For example, the American Diabetes Association recommends a 500-750 kcal/day energy deficit coupled with regular physical activity. Dietitians follow this approach and recommend eating 4-6 small meals throughout the day.

Does the portion-control strategy work in the long-run? Rarely. A cohort study with a 9-year follow-up from the United Kingdom on 176,495 obese individuals indicated that only 3,528 of them succeeded in attaining normal body weight by the end of the study. That is a failure rate of 98%!

Intermittent fasting is not constant caloric restriction. Restricting calories causes a compensatory increase in hunger and worse, a decrease in the body's metabolic rate, a double curse! Because when we are burning fewer calories per day, it becomes increasingly harder to lose weight and much easier to gain weight back after we have lost it. This type of diet puts the body into a "starvation mode" as metabolism revs down to conserve energy.

Intermittent fasting does not have any of these drawbacks.

Health Benefits Of Intermittent Fasting

- Increases metabolism leading to weight and body fat loss: Unlike a daily caloric reduction diet, intermittent fasting raises metabolism. This makes sense from a survival standpoint. If we do not eat, the body uses stored energy as fuel so that we can stay alive to find another meal. Hormones allow the body to switch energy sources from food to body fat.

Studies demonstrate this phenomenon clearly. For example, four days of continuous fasting increased Basal Metabolic Rate by 12%. Levels of the neurotransmitter norepinephrine, which prepares the body for action, increased by 117%. Fatty acids in the bloodstream increased over 370% as the body switched from burning food to burning stored fats.

- No loss in muscle mass: Unlike a constant calorie-restriction diet, intermittent fasting does not burn muscles as many have feared. In 2010, researchers looked at a group of subjects who underwent 70 days of alternate daily fasting (ate one day and fasted the next). Their muscle mass started off at 52.0 kg and ended at 51.9 kg. In other words, there was no loss of muscles but they did lose 11.4%

of fat and saw major improvements in LDL cholesterol and triglyceride levels.

During fasting, the body naturally produces more human growth hormone to preserve lean muscles and bones. Muscle mass is generally preserved until body fat drops below 4%. Therefore, most people are not at risk of muscle-wasting when doing intermittent fasting.

Reverses insulin resistance, type 2 diabetes, and fatty liver

Type 2 diabetes is a condition whereby there is simply too much sugar in the body, to the point that the cells can no longer respond to insulin and take in any more glucose from the blood (insulin resistance), resulting in high blood sugar. Also, the liver becomes loaded with fat as it tries to clear out the excess glucose by converting it to and storing it as fat.

Therefore, to reverse this condition, two things have to happen -

- First, stop putting more sugar into the body.
- Second, burn the remaining sugar off.

The best diet to achieve this is a low-carbohydrate, moderate-protein, and high-healthy fat diet, also called ketogentic diet. (Remember that carbohydrate raises blood sugar the most, protein to some degree, and fat the least.) That is why a low-carb diet will help reduce the burden of incoming glucose. For some people, this is already enough to reverse insulin resistance and type 2 diabetes. However, in more severe cases, diet alone is not sufficient.

What about exercise? Exercise will help burn off glucose in the skeletal muscles but not all the tissues and organs, including the fatty liver. Clearly, exercise is important, but to eliminate the excess glucose in the organs, there is the need to temporarily "starve" the cells.

Intermittent fasting can accomplish this. That is why historically, people called fasting a cleanse or a detox. It can be a very powerful tool to get rid of all the excesses. It is the fastest way to lower blood glucose and insulin levels, and eventually reversing insulin resistance, type 2 diabetes, and fatty liver.

By the way, taking insulin for type 2 diabetes does not address the root cause of the problem, which is excess sugar in the body. It is true that insulin will drive the glucose away from the blood, resulting in lower blood glucose, but where does the sugar go? The liver is just going to turn it all into fat, fat in the liver and fat in the abdomen. Patients who go on insulin often end up gaining more weight, which worsens their diabetes.

- Enhances heart health: Overtime, high blood glucose from type 2 diabetes can damage the blood vessels and nerves that control the heart. The longer one has diabetes, the higher the chances that heart disease will develop. By lowering blood sugar through intermittent fasting, the risk of cardiovascular disease and stroke is also reduced. In addition, intermittent fasting has been shown to improve blood pressure, total and LDL (bad) cholesterol, blood triglycerides, and inflammatory markers associated with many chronic diseases.

- Boosts brain power: Multiple studies demonstrated fasting has many neurologic benefits including attention and focus, reaction time, immediate memory, cognition, and generation of new brain cells. Mice studies also showed that intermittent fasting reduces brain inflammation and prevents the symptoms of Alzheimer's.

What To Expect With Intermittent Fasting

Hunger Goes Down

We normally feel hunger pangs about four hours after a meal. So if we fast for 24 hours, does it mean that our hunger sensations will be six times more severe? Of course not.

Many people are concerned that fasting will result in extreme hunger and overeating. Studies showed that on the day after a one-day fast, there is, indeed, a 20% increase in caloric intake. However, with repeated fasting, hunger and appetite surprisingly decrease.

Hunger comes in waves. If we do nothing, the hunger dissipates after a while. Drinking tea (all kinds) or coffee (with or without caffeine) is often enough to fight it off. However, it is best to drink it black though a teaspoon or two of cream or half-and-half will not trigger much insulin response. Do not use any types of sugar or artificial sweeteners. If necessary, bone broth can also be taken during fasting.

Blood sugar does not crash

Sometimes people worry that blood sugar will fall very low during fasting and they will become shaky and sweaty. This does not actually happen as blood sugar is tightly monitored by the body and there are multiple mechanisms to keep it in the proper range. During fasting, the body begins to break down glycogen in the liver to release glucose. This happens every night during our sleep.

If we fast for longer than 24-36 hours, glycogen stores become depleted and the liver will manufacture new glucose using glycerol which is a by-product of the breakdown of fat (a process called gluconeogenesis). Apart from using glucose, our brain cells can also use ketones for energy. Ketones are produced when fat is metabolized and they can supply up to 75% of the brain's energy requirements (the other 25% from glucose).

The only exception is for those who are taking diabetic medications and insulin. You MUST first consult your doctor as the dosages will probably need to be reduced while you are fasting. Otherwise, if you overmedicate and hypoglycemia develops, which can be dangerous, you must have some sugar to reverse it. This will break the fast and make it counterproductive.

The Dawn Phenomenon

After a period of fasting, especially in the morning, some people experience high blood glucose. This dawn phenomenon is a result of the circadian rhythm whereby just before awakening, the body secretes higher levels of

several hormones to prepare for the
upcoming day -

- Adrenaline - to give the body
  some energy
- Growth hormone - to help repair
  and make new protein
- Glucagon - to move glucose from
  storage in the liver to the blood
  for use as energy
- Cortisol, the stress hormone - to
  activate the body

These hormones peak in the morning
hours, then fall to lower levels during
the day. In non-diabetics, the magnitude
of the blood sugar rise is small and most
people will not even notice it. However,
for the majority of the diabetics, there
can be a noticeable spike in blood
glucose as the liver dumps sugar into
the blood.

This will happen in extended fasts too. When there is no food, insulin levels stay low while the liver releases some of its stored sugar and fat. This is natural and not a bad thing at all. The magnitude of the spike will decrease as the liver becomes less bloated with sugar and fat.

Who Should Not Do Intermittent Fasting?

- Women who want to get pregnant, are pregnant, or are breastfeeding.
- Those who are malnourished or underweight.
- Children under 18 years of age and elders.
- Those who have gout.
- Those who have gastroesophageal reflux disease (GERD).

- Those who have eating disorders should first consult with their doctors.
- Those who are taking diabetic medications and insulin must first consult with their doctors as dosages will need to be reduced.
- Those who are taking medications should first consult with their doctors as the timing of medications may be affected.
- Those who feel very stressed or have cortisol issues should not fast because fasting is another stressor.
- Those who are training very hard most days of the week should not fast.
- How To Prepare For Intermittent Fasting?

If anyone is thinking about starting intermittent fasting, it is best to first switch to a low-carbohydrate, high-healthy fat diet for three weeks. This will allow the body to become accustomed to using fat rather than glucose as a source of energy. That means getting rid of all sugars, grains (bread, cookies, pastries, pasta, rice), legumes, and refined vegetable oils. This will minimize most side effects associated with fasting.

Start with a shorter fast of 16 hours, for example, from dinner (8 pm) until lunch (12 pm) the next day. You can eat normally between 12 pm and 8 pm, and you can eat either two or three meals. Once you feel comfortable with it, you can extend the fast to 18, 20 hours.

For shorter fasts, you can do it everyday, continuously. For more extended fasts, such as 24-36 hours, you can do it 1-3 times a week, alternating between fasting and normal eating days.

There is no single fasting regimen that is correct. The key is to choose one that works best for you. Some people achieve results with shorter fasts, others may need longer fasts. Some people do a classic water-only fast, others do a tea and coffee fast, still others a bone broth fast. No matter what you do, it is very important to stay hydrated and monitor yourself. If you feel ill at any point, you should stop immediately. You can be hungry, but you should not feel sick.

THE MIDDLE AGE SPREAD

Most women gain weight as they age, but excess pounds aren't inevitable. To minimize menopause weight gain, step up your activity level and enjoy a healthy diet.

As you get older, you might notice that maintaining your usual weight becomes more difficult. In fact, many women gain weight around the menopause transition.

Menopause weight gain isn't inevitable, however. You can reverse course by paying attention to healthy-eating habits and leading an active lifestyle.

WHAT CAUSES MENOPAUSE WEIGHT GAIN?

The hormonal changes of menopause might make you more likely to gain weight around your abdomen than around your hips and thighs. But, hormonal changes alone don't necessarily cause menopause weight gain. Instead, the weight gain is usually related to aging, as well as lifestyle and genetic factors.

For example, muscle mass typically diminishes with age, while fat increases. Losing muscle mass slows the rate at which your body uses calories (metabolism). This can make it more challenging to maintain a healthy weight. If you continue to eat as you always have and don't increase your physical activity, you're likely to gain weight.

Genetic factors might also play a role in menopause weight gain. If your parents or other close relatives carry extra weight around the abdomen, you're likely to do the same.

Other factors, such as a lack of exercise, unhealthy eating and not enough sleep, might contribute to menopause weight gain. When people don't get enough sleep, they tend to snack more and consume more calories.

HOW RISKY IS WEIGHT GAIN AFTER MENOPAUSE?

Menopause weight gain can have serious implications for your health. Excess weight, especially around your midsection, increases your risk of many issues, including:

- Breathing problems

- Heart and blood vessel disease

- Type 2 diabetes

Excess weight also increases your risk of various types of cancer, including breast, colon and endometrial cancers.

WHAT'S THE BEST WAY TO PREVENT WEIGHT GAIN AFTER MENOPAUSE?

There's no magic formula for preventing — or reversing — menopause weight gain. Simply stick to weight-control basics:

• Move more. Physical activity, including aerobic exercise and strength training, can help you shed excess pounds and maintain a healthy weight. As you gain muscle, your body burns calories more efficiently — which makes it easier to control your weight.

For most healthy adults, experts recommend moderate aerobic activity, such as brisk walking, for at least 150 minutes a week or vigorous aerobic activity, such as jogging, for at least 75 minutes a week.

In addition, strength training exercises are recommended at least twice a week. If you want to lose weight or meet specific fitness goals, you might need to exercise more.

• Eat less. To maintain your current weight — let alone lose excess pounds — you might need about 200 fewer calories a day during your 50s than you did during your 30s and 40s.

To reduce calories without skimping on nutrition, pay attention to what you're eating and drinking. Choose more fruits, vegetables and whole grains, particularly those that are less processed and contain more fiber.

In general, a plant-based diet is healthier than other options. Legumes, nuts, soy, fish and low-fat dairy products are good choices. Meat, such as red meat, or chicken, should be eaten in limited quantities. Replace butter, stick margarine and shortening with oils, such as olive or vegetable oil.

• Check your sweet habit. Added sugars account for nearly 300 calories a day in the average American diet. About half of these calories come from sugar-sweetened beverages, such as soft drinks, juices, energy drinks, flavored waters, and sweetened coffee and tea.

Other foods that contribute to excess dietary sugar include cookies, pies, cakes, doughnuts, ice cream and candy.

• Limit alcohol. Alcoholic beverages add excess calories to your diet and increase the risk of gaining weight.

• Seek support. Surround yourself with friends and loved ones who support your efforts to eat a healthy diet and increase your physical activity. Better yet, team up and make the lifestyle changes together.

Remember, successful weight loss at any stage of life requires permanent changes in diet and exercise habits. Commit to lifestyle changes and enjoy a healthier you.

BALANCING HORMONES AND CRESCENDO FASTING

Women are naturally more sensitive to intermittent fasting, most likely due to the presence of a chemical named kisspeptin. This sensitivity can cause abnormal periods, disturb the normal cycles, making women hormonally unbalanced.

That being said, it is vital to keep in mind that no two women are exactly the same. There are some who do great with intermittent fasting, and others don't. Should this mean that intermittent fasting is not meant for those who are sensitive to it? No.

For such women, it is preferable to try a gentler version of fasting called the Crescendo fasting. Crescendo fasting has proven itself to be the perfect method for middle-aged women over 50 who are unable to follow other IF routines and generally find it harder to lose weight.

Following is an example to follow a crescendo fasting:

• Perform intermittent fasting twice a week, preferably on non-consecutive days (E.g., Tuesday and Saturday) fasting for 12-14 hours.

• Perform light physical activities on the fasting days, for example, gentle walking, light yoga, or light aerobic exercises

• Add another fast day after two weeks of IF (E.g., Tuesday, Thursday, and Saturday)

THE PHASE ONE DIET FOR MAXIMUM FAT BURNING

There may be a lot of readers who are only familiar with one or the other. Both have a unique style that packs a big punch to fat loss and proper health. On the surface only one of them is considered a "diet," but even that term is held very loosely. I am very familiar with both of them in regards to fat loss and overall health benefits so to give an overall summary for both will be suitable. I truly believe that if you bridge the gap and combine these two styles, you will be able to produce some pretty amazing fat loss results. Let's begin!

FASTING FOR FAT LOSS IS EXTREMELY EFFECTIVE

The idea of fasting in a diet plan tends to get very negative remarks within the fitness culture. Many companies and trainers have us believing that if you aren't eating every few hours than your metabolism will slow down or cause our bodies to go into "starvation mode." Before we go any further, we must establish that "slowing of the metabolism" may be one of the biggest myths in the entire fitness industry. Metabolism is decreased under chronic, low-calorie consumptions that last weeks on end. This does not happen when fasting is done a couple times a week. Here is a simple outline of how intermittent fasting is implemented into someone's schedule. I'll explain how this can be tweaked to your liking later.

1. Eat normal until dinner (2-4 meals, not 6-8)
2. Eat your dinner but stop eating after that.
3. Fast until dinner the following day. (No calorie consumption)
4. For that meal just eat a regular size dinner.

In this approach you are still fasting for a 24-hour period, but are still having a meal every day. This is done typically 1-2 times a week. If you need to drop a lot of weight before a vacation or reunion, then you can fast 3 times a week. I would only recommend this for a few weeks.

What You Learn About Yourself During Fasting

When fasting, you will want to take note of any changes in the way you eat. Once you have completed a 24 hour fast a few times, the reasons of what, when, and why you eat may be revealed to you. A lot of the reasons why we eat is because of emotional connections or pure habit and not with actual hunger itself. Sometimes we are so conditioned to eat at certain times that we consume a meal when we aren't hungry.

Intermittent Fasting Is A Lifestyle And Not A Diet

The reason why it is not considered a "diet" is because it doesn't restrict you to certain foods, recipes, combinations, instructions, or charts to follow in order to lose weight. It rids you of obsessive compulsive eating habits and allows you variety. Instead of completely avoiding a particular food because someone told you to, adding a variety of foods will actually prevent you from over-eating any type of "bad" food. Now that we have established this area of fat loss, let's turn to a deeper issue in regards to diet and health.

What Is the Phase One Diet AKA The Fungus Link?

Doug Kaufmann is the mastermind behind the idea of fungus and yeast contributing to bad health and weight loss failures. He has researched and documented how fungi produces poisonous substances called "mycotoxins" which causes many health problems. He tackles the problem by addressing areas where fungi and yeast can enter the body, but also provides the solution in starving the fungus to reverse the symptoms of so many health problems in America. He has found that fungi, like people, crave specific carbohydrates. Knowing that fungi must have carbohydrates in order to thrive inside the body makes the Phase 1 Diet understandable to use.

So What Is Allowed On the Phase 1 Diet?

This is the only "diet" that I would ever recommend that actually restricts certain types of food, but for a specific reason. The exclusion of certain foods is done momentarily to starve and kill the fungus as well as exposing the root of food cravings. Food cravings that are not under control can be detrimental to your health as well as the added pounds on the belly, thighs, hips, you name it.

Fungus overgrowth may in fact be the root failure in losing the weight. As long as you are addicted to certain foods you will continue to eat and eat mindlessly. Many people find that their health elevates to a level where they can't believe how great they feel. A large reason for this is because of the specific food choice that starves and prevents overgrowth of fungus. Many people are living better because of this break through approach to eating. Here is a quick outline of food choices that are acceptable on the Phase 1 Diet.

Example of Acceptable Foods For The Phase 1 Diet

1)Eggs

2)FRUIT: Berries, Grapefruit, Lemon, Lime, Green Apples, Avocado, Fresh Coconut

3)MEATS: Virtually all meat including fish, poultry and beef

4)VEGETABLES: Fresh, unblemished vegetables and freshly made vegetable juice

5)BEVERAGES: Bottled or filtered water, non-fruity herbal teas, stevia sweetened fresh lemonade, freshly squeezed carrot juice.

6)VINEGAR: apple cider vinegar

7)OILS: olive, grape, flax seed, cold pressed virgin coconut oil

8)NUTS: raw nuts, including pecans, almonds, walnuts, cashews, and pumpkin seeds. Stored nuts tend to gather mold, so be careful!

9)SWEETENERS: Stevia, Xylitol

10)DAIRY: Organic Butter, Organic Yogurt, (use the following very sparingly) cream cheese, unsweetened whipping cream, real sour cream.

Note: Once again these food choices are only allowed during the very beginning of the diet. After awhile you are allowed to introduce more and more varieties of food, but only once the fungus overgrowth is taken care of. There a couple of phases that he has constructed so you aren't left clueless what to do next. Remember, restriction of certain foods is only for a short period of time. I truly believe that if you begin this diet in conjunction with intermittent fasting, it will remove all the guesswork out of fat loss. Losing weight is nothing more than burning more calories than what you are consuming. Intermittent fasting creates the huge calorie deficit while the Phase 1 Diet breaks food addictions that cause people to be overweight and succumb to health problems caused by fungus.

AUTOPHAGY

Autophagy means "self-eating" — but rest assured, this is a good thing. Autophagy is the method by which your body cleans out damaged cells and toxins, helping you regenerate newer, healthier cells.

Over time, our cells accumulate a variety of dead organelles, damaged proteins and oxidized particles that clog the body's inner workings. This accelerates the effects of aging and age-related diseases because cells aren't able to divide and function normally.

Because many of our cells, like those in the brain, need to last a lifetime, the body developed a unique way of ridding itself of those faulty parts and defending itself naturally against disease. Enter: autophagy.

HOW AUTOPHAGY WORKS

Think of your body as a kitchen. After making a meal, you clean up the counter, throw away the leftovers and recycle some of the food. The next day, you have a clean kitchen. This is autophagy doing its thing in your body, and doing it well.

Now, think of the same scenario, but you're older and not as efficient. After making your meal, you leave remnants on the counter. Some of it gets into the garbage, some of it doesn't. The scraps linger on the counter, garbage and recycling bin. They never make it out the door to the dumpster, and toxic waste starts to build up in your kitchen. There's food fermentation on the floor and all kinds of nasty smells wafting out the door.

Due to the onslaught of pollutants and toxins, you're having a hard time keeping up with the daily grime. This scenario resembles autophagy that isn't working as well as it should.

Autophagy usually hums along ⬚uietly behind the scenes in maintenance mode. It plays a role in the way your body responds to periods of stress, maintains balance and regulates cellular function.

There's evidence that when you trigger autophagy, you slow down the aging process, reduce inflammation and boost your overall performance. To help your body resist disease and support longevity, you can increase your autophagy response naturally (more on that later).

AUTOPHAGY AND LONGEVITY

Humans evolved to live longer because of our ability to respond to biological stressors, from physical activity to famine. A study from Newcastle University study found that this ability is due to small adaptations in a protein known as p62 that induces autophagy.

By sensing the metabolic byproducts that cause cell damage (called reactive oxygen species ROS), protein p62 activates to induce autophagy, or start cleaning. Specifically, p62 proteins remove all the damaged goods that have accumulated in your body so that you're better euipped to handle biological stress. Homeostasis (balanced cellular function) and vibrant health are a direct result of p62 protein doing its thing during autophagy. As a result, the damaged goods that build up in your body over time are turned over for new cell formation — and this is what keeps you healthy.

While humans possess this capacity, lower organisms like fruit flies do not. So, the research team set about identifying the part of human protein p62 that allows for the sensing of ROS. They then created genetically modified fruit flies with "humanized" p62. The result? The "humanized" flies survived longer in stressful conditions.

"This tells us that abilities, like sensing stress and activating protective processes like autophagy, may have evolved to allow better stress resistance and a longer lifespan," says the study's lead author Dr. Viktor Korolchuk.

The process sounds good, but how do you really benefit from autophagy?

BENEFITS OF AUTOPHAGY

We're just beginning to understand how autophagy works in the body, and what we know so far is primarily based on rodent studies. Mice aren't humans, but the evidence is compelling:

• May control inflammation, slow down the aging process and protect against neurodegenerative disease.

• May help fight infection and support immunity.

• Triggering autophagy might help you live longer.

HOW TO INCREASE AUTOPHAGY

There are several ways you can turn up your body's autophagy process (that have nothing to do with juice cleanses). To cleanse your cells and reduce inflammation, and generally keep your body running in tip-top shape, take these five simple steps to increase the autophagy process.

Keep in mind that because autophagy is a response to stress, you need to trick your body into thinking it's a little bit under siege. Here's how:

1. EAT A HIGH-FAT, LOW-CARB DIET

Whittel stresses the importance of eating fat to activate autophagy. "Fat needs to be the dominant macronutrient in our diets because it's different from protein. Whereas protein can turn into a carb and become a sugar, [fat cannot]," she says.

Specifically, a keto diet gives you an edge when it comes to autophagy. The shift from burning glucose (carbs) to ketones (fats) mimics what occurs naturally in a fasted state — and this may increase autophagy in its own right.

2. GO ON A PROTEIN FAST

Once or twice a week, limit your protein consumption to 15-25 grams a day. This gives your body a full day to recycle proteins, which will help reduce inflammation and cleanse your cells without any muscle loss. During this time, while autophagy gets triggered, your body is forced to consume its own proteins and toxins.

3. PRACTICE INTERMITTENT FASTING

Research suggests that fasting increases autophagy. How long to fast for autophagy? In a 2010 study, mice fasted for 24 or 48 hours to promote autophagy. It's not clear how that translates to humans (yet), but we do know that intermittent fasting is associated with weight loss, insulin sensitivity and lower disease risk.

4. EXERCISE

Another reason to hit the gym: in human and rodent studies, exercise has been shown to stimulate autophagy. In a 2018 study, 12 men completed an eight-week exercise program consisting of continuous state cycling or high-intensity interval cycling for three days per week. The researchers concluded that both styles of training supported autophagy, which supports the idea that all movement is good movement.

Whittel emphasizes a "less is more" approach to exercise for inducing autophagy and favors high-intensity interval training (HIIT). "Weightlifting and resistance training exercises for 30 minutes every other day is the best way to activate autophagy. It's about getting in that short-term, acute stress, because autophagy loves the stress of interval training." Whittel applies interval training to her walks by alternating between a brisk and slow pace.

5. GET RESTORATIVE SLEEP

You can reap the benefits of autophagy while you're asleep too, says Whittel. A 2016 rodent study suggests that autophagy follows circadian rhythms, and sleep fragmentation — or short interruptions of sleep — seems to disrupt autophagy. Want to feel your best and maybe live longer?

What is nutrient timing?

Consuming the right nutrients is incredibly important for meeting your health and fitness goals. Not eating the right balance of nutrients can lead to fat gain, muscle loss and reduced athletic performance.

But how about the timing of nutrients? Should you eat your key performance nutrients before or after exercise, and how long before or after? And how much should you eat at a time?

Nutrient timing has been a hot topic for a number of years. The general consensus used to be:

- Eat high carb performance meals post-workout.
- Eat low carb meals the rest of the time.

This was based on a solid theory. Protein prevents muscle breakdown, and carbohydrates replenish your glycogen stores, which are depleted during workouts. Getting a good dose of carbs and protein after a workout should help you recover more ⬚uickly, and boost muscle synthesis right when your body is working its hardest to rebuild your muscles.

However, this was based on some limited science.

Firstly, they didn't consider final outcomes. What I mean by this, is things you actually are aiming for, such as improved performance, fat loss, or muscle gain. The studies instead were primarily concerned with protein synthesis rates and glycogen replenishment rates. It's a nice theory that these will lead to improved performance and body composition, but there's no guarantee they do.

Secondly, they were short studies. What's most important, is what happens in the long term.

So, what have we learned in recent years?

Well, studies have shown that if you don't consume carbs after working out, but instead just eat carbs throughout the day, you will replenish glycogen stores in about 24 hours. If you consume carbs right after workout, glycogen replacement will be faster.

This means that if you exercise more than once a day, consuming carbs right after exercise is beneficial.

But if you exercise hard no more than once a day, it doesn't matter much when you eat.

Nutrient Timing For Muscle Growth

For years the prevailing wisdom was that you had to drink a protein shake as soon as you finished a workout to get maximum benefit.

However, a growing amount of evidence suggests that this simply isn't the case.

A large analysis carried out in 2013 went looking for all studies conducted to date which were investigating just how important timing was for muscle hypertrophy and strength improvements. They found that, on average, there was no relationship.

However, there is a time when the old advice of eating a big pile of carbs and protein right after a workout does apply. In a massive review of all the evidence, published in the Journal of the International Society of Sports Nutrition, the authors came to the conclusion that if you haven't eaten for

3-4 hours before working out, your body enters a catabolic where muscle synthesis is reduced. In these circumstances, a large protein shake after a workout is an excellent idea to push your body into an anabolic or muscle building state.

When should you eat your daily calories?

There is little evidence that there is any difference between someone who eats 2500 calorie in 3 meals, compared to someone who eats 2500 calories in 4 or 5 meals.

There have been studies that have shown that eating more meals a day tends to correlate with obesity. However, this is simply because people who eat more meals tend to eat more food in general. If you eat the same number of calories spread out over more meals, it makes no difference.

Another common belief is that eating just before going to bed can lead to gaining body fat.

This idea has stuck around as it seems to be true that people who eat more in the evening are in general less healthy. However, people that eat late tend to eat more food overall, and eat less healthily. When total calorie consumption and food quality is accounted for, the evening effect disappears.

Eating regular meals does help stave off hunger and prevent you from making poor food choices. One study showed that skipping breakfast meant that participants were more hungry during the day, so snacked on unhealthy food and ended up eating more calories.

If you find yourself snacking on sweets and unhealthy snacks throughout the day, consider eating regular meals of wholesome, non-calorie dense foods, like green vegetables instead.

Intermittent fasting has been shown to result in an improvement in body composition for many people.

The reasons why this works is a little unclear at present, as not much research has been done on the topic.

It has been shown that restricting your eating to a window of 8 hours a day has significant positive effects on some health-related hormones, which may aid body composition.

It is also likely that restricting you eating to a short window simply means you eat fewer calories.

It has also been shown that if you exercise when fasted, you burn fat more readily than someone who has eaten recently. This suggests that if you fast, your body goes into a fat burning state, making it easier to burn fat. The jury is still out on this effect though, as some studies have shown no effect on overall body fat.

When should you eat for improved athletic performance?

If you're looking to get that extra boost of energy during a workout or a race, is it best to eat just before exercising, or several hours before?

You would expect there to be the ideal time before exercise to get your calories. But surprisingly, studies have shown that for exercise lasting less than an hour, so long as you eat adequate calories at some point during the day, it doesn't seem to matter much when you eat them.

However, where timing does become important is when preparing for a workout or race of longer than 90 minutes. If you're planning on running or cycling at moderate to high intensity for more than an hour and a half, carb loading can improve performance and push back the onset of fatigue.

Over the course of 90 minutes, your body can simply run out of energy. Carb loading is where you consume an elevated level of carbohydrates in the days approaching an event, to increase your energy stores. This has been shown to improve performance.

To get the maximum benefit, you need to eat carbohydrates with a low glycemic index such as pasta and grains in the days running up to the event, then switch to faster burning carbs such as sugars in the hours before the race.

In conclusion

Nutrient timing is important for some people, especially athletes, people who exercise multiple times a day or for over 2 hours at a time. For these people, getting a decent amount of calories in the form of carbs and protein can improve performance and aid recovery.

If you've just done a hard workout, you don't have to have a massive meal right away, unless you haven't eaten for 3-4 hours prior to working out. If this is the case, try to eat something as soon as possible, as this will help muscle synthesis.

If you're trying to lose fat, consider trying intermittent fasting. It doesn't work for everyone, but it has been revolutionary for others. For most people, nutrient timing is not a significantly important issue. It's much more important to pay attention to what you eat, and how much you eat, rather than when you eat.

HOW TO BREAK YOUR INTERMITTENT FAST

• It is very rare for individuals to experience distress while following intermittent fasting protocols

• Sometimes people struggle with gastrointestinal issues while ending extended fasting protocols

• Certain foods like eggs and nuts can be problematic when consumed during your breakfast meal

• Follow our proven strategies to help prevent and ease the potential side effects of breaking your fast

• For most, gastric distress usually go away within two-to-four weeks of staying consistent with your fasting schedule

Individuals who are following intermittent fasting or time restricted eating (TRE) strategies usually don't encounter issues while ending their fasts shorter than 24 hours. However, some people can develop gastrointestinal issues during their "breakfast" meals while doing longer periods of fasting.

The definition of the word breakfast is the first meal of the day and its origin was derived from the late Middle English verbs "break" and "fast." The word literally means to break the fasting period from the day before. It does not mean to make sure you fill your bellies within minutes of waking. No matter what time you eat after a night's sleep is your breakfast whether it is 5:00 am or 5:00 pm because it is when you break your fast.

Most individuals have no problems ending common intermittent fasting protocols, such as the 16, 18 or 24 hour fast. It's usually when people start following the alternate daily 36 or 42 hour protocols, or start extended fasting where they may encounter tummy troubles.

In my experience, not everyone struggles to end their fast. Some people can eat almost anything they like when they break their fasts and feel perfectly normal. Occasionally, an individual who has never experienced issues breaking their fast before may suddenly start to experience trouble. Don't be discouraged. This isn't uncommon and doesn't mean something is wrong. Each fast is different. Your body is different. Be patient and more mindful the next time you go to break your fast.

TROUBLE ENDING YOUR FAST:

During fasting, production of digestive enzymes slows, which may cause some gastrointestinal distress when you start to eat again. For example, you may experience:

- Diarrhea or loose stools

- Gas pains and bloating

- Nausea and vomiting (rare)

WHAT FOODS TO AVOID WHEN YOU BREAK YOUR FAST?

It usually takes your digestive system two-to-four weeks to adapt to fasting. Until then, you might want to avoid eating these foods during your breakfast meal:

• Eggs

• Nuts and nut butters

• Seeds and seed butters

• Raw vegetables and leafy greens (cooked are fine)

• Dairy products (butter is fine)

• Red meats

• Alcohol

Not everyone is sensitive to all or any of these foods. If that's not you, then don't worry. Eat all the eggs and almonds you want after a fast. Have that big steak! Enjoy!

But if you are having problems, try to eliminate these food items from your breakfast. Most people are able to resume eating them during their second post-fast meal without difficulty.

FIVE STEP BREAKFAST PROTOCOL

If you are finding yourself spending too much time in your bathroom when you end your intermittent or extended fast, then try to follow this protocol:

1. Add one tablespoon of psyllium husk to one cup of water, and let sit 5-10 minutes. It will get very thick and jelly-like. Drink 15 to 30 minutes prior to eating. This insoluble fibre helps the gut get working again.

2. Start your meal off with a cup of tomato and cucumber salad with some chopped parsley. You can add a tablespoon of extra virgin olive oil if you like.

3. To play it safe and keep your protein sources to poultry or fish. They can be cooked in fat and poultry skin can be consumed. Try to limit your protein

intake to the size and thickness of the palm of your hand.

4. Fill the rest of your plate with non-starchy, above-ground vegetables that have been cooked in healthy fats, like avocado or coconut oil, butter or ghee.

5. Finish your meal off with an avocado if you're still feeling hungry.

If you follow this protocol and still experience problems, try to take another tablespoon of psyllium husk in a cup of water. The next time you are fasting and are about to resume eating, you may want to try the above protocol but add in two tablespoons of psyllium in water at the start.

It usually takes about two-to-four weeks for individuals doing intermittent fasting to stop experiencing discomfort while ending their fasts. Those who practice extended fasting often also notice an improvement usually three or four fasts down the road. Hang in there. It does get easier!

THE MYTHS

Intermittent fasting has become widely popular. Both men and women of all age ranges have jumped on the bandwagon of this health and fitness trend to help them lose weight and improve their health. Before you go following in the steps of supposed fans, you want to be sure that you are clear on what this type of "diet" really consists of.

According to Dr. Robert Zembroski although fasting has been said to be good for the mind and body, there are also things that you should watch out for when you're done.

"Those that fast often indulge in eating high-calorie high-fat foods with the perception that fasting will allow them to devour whatever they want," he said. "When you deprive the body of food, there is a physiological drive to overeat due to the release of appetite hormones including ghrelin and leptin and excitation of the hunger center in your brain. This will cause people to overeat after their fast."

To help you along your journey, here are 10 myths — debunked — about intermittent fasting.

MYTH: YOU CAN EAT AS MUCH AS YOU WANT WHEN YOU STOP YOUR FAST.

You should still be eating regular sized meals.

Intermittent fasting — and any other diet you decide to go on — is just the start of your healthier lifestyle. Unfortunately, though, many believe that they can go back to uncontrolled eating once they've ended their fast. And, according to Dr. Mike Roussell, co-founder of Neuro Coffee, doing this will basically be counterproductive to all the work you've put in.

"The key to being successful with I.F. is that you need to eat as you normally would when you end your fast," he said. "If you fast all day until dinner, but then eat a dinner that is the size of breakfast/lunch/dinner, it negates the time that you spent fasting."

MYTH: FASTING WILL SLOW YOUR METABOLISM DOWN.

You should not be restricting calories.

Whether in fear or anticipation of slowing your metabolism down through intermittent fasting, Blum says that this is actually a myth and he's here to debunk it.

"Intermittent fasting isn't to calorie restrict; it's restricting the time in which calories are consumed," he said. "Waiting a few extra hours to eat your first meal will not make a difference in metabolic rate. Changes in metabolic occur with undereating — which should not be happening when on an intermittent fasting diet."

MYTH: FASTING IS BETTER THAN SNACKING FOR WEIGHT LOSS.

It depends on the calories of the snack.

When dieting, it is often said that you should be snacking between each meal. One of the main myths about intermittent fasting, however, makes those who try it think that it should be a substitute for healthy snacking.

"In the end, weight loss comes down to a constant calorie deficit," Blum told INSIDER. "It doesn't matter if those calories are spread throughout the day or consumed in a four to eight hour period. Do what is best is for your body and lifestyle to reach the goals that are set."

MYTH: YOU'RE GOING TO LOSE WEIGHT NO MATTER WHAT.

Weight loss is not guaranteed.

Contrary to popular belief, intermittent fasting — or fasting in general — does not always lead to weight loss. It doesn't matter how long the fast is for if you're breaking the fast by throwing down burgers, pizza, and candy, results are going to be slim to none. I.F. works hand-in-hand with a healthy diet. Each fasting period cannot be treated like a cheat day for the diet to work.

MYTH: FASTING FOR WEIGHT LOSS WORKS BETTER THAN OTHER WEIGHT LOSS STRATEGIES.

All calorie restriction will lead to weight loss.

If you're under the impression that intermittent fasting is the best option for losing weight, you may want to think again.

"Intermittent fasting at the most basic level is an exercise in caloric restriction," Roussell said. "Intermittent fasting has not been shown to work better than other means and methods for losing weight."

MYTH: WORKING OUT IS IMPOSSIBLE IF YOU'RE FASTING.

Working out while fasting is possible.

Actually the best time to work out is on an empty stomach first thing in the morning. That way you'll be burning the fat already stored on your body instead of the calories from what you've just consumed. Eat your breakfast after your workout to replenish your body.

MYTH: EATING A BIG BREAKFAST IS A NECESSITY SINCE IT'S CONSIDERED THE MOST IMPORTANT MEAL OF THE DAY.

Eat what works for your body.

Though you're told you should be consuming a good amount for breakfast to fuel your day, the way we're lead to believe is not necessarily true.

This is a big part of American culture —
the big, complete breakfast. Of course,
cereal companies want you to think that,
but really, you can listen to your body
and have a small breakfast (since most
people don't have much of an appetite
when they wake up). Then, you can eat
a substantial lunch — especially if
you've worked out in the morning or
skipped breakfast altogether. You can
choose whichever meal you want to be
your biggest meal of the day. It's all
about what works for your body and
your lifestyle.

MYTH: YOU'LL BECOME EXTREMELY HEALTHY AND FIT BY FASTING.

Fasting won't do much overnight.

Intermittent fasting — when combined
with proper exercise and care — can
assist you in losing weight, but we must
caution those who are considering the
diet to know that doing it by itself is not

a magical way to be successful at becoming fit.

There is no magic bullet solution. Health and fitness are things that you have to work to maintain throughout your entire life — don't take them for granted. Fasting won't give you your ideal body overnight and if you do lose weight, you will have to continue maintaining it with healthy habits, which includes a nutritious diet and regular exercise.

MYTH: ALL INTERMITTENT FASTING IS THE SAME AND EVERYONE GETS THE SAME RESULTS.

Everyone's body will respond to fasting differently.

There is no "official" definition regarding what intermittent fasting is. And, there are several types. Some I.F. protocols are fasting every other day entirely, while others are ingesting a certain amount of kcals or doing time-restricted feeding to a six, eight, or 10 hour window day to day.

MYTH: INTERMITTENT FASTING WORKS BECAUSE YOUR BODY DOESN'T PROCESS FOODS AT NIGHT.

If you eat at 3 a.m., rest assured, your body will digest it.

One huge misconception about fasting is the reason why it works. Though it's often thought that digestion doesn't occur after a certain time, this myth is not true.

Your body will digest food no matter what time it is. It's a matter of allowing your body a significant time (whether experts agree on 12-16-18 hours remains unseen) to focus on other metabolic processes like autophagy and cellular repair, instead of diverting attention to digestion. If you eat at 3 a.m., rest assured, your body will digest it. Truthfully, I'm a terrible candidate for

I.F. I have a robust Latin late night dinner plan culture and early morning workouts that I physically will pass out during if I don't eat breakfast. I also physically cannot sleep if I go to bed too late without eating. Here I am, however, a living and breathing testament.

WEIGHT LOSS TIPS FOR AFTER 50s

For many people, maintaining a healthy weight or losing excess body fat can become harder as the years go by.

Unhealthy habits, a mostly sedentary lifestyle, poor dietary choices, and metabolic changes can all contribute to weight gain after the age of 50.

However, with a few simple adjustments, you can lose weight at any age — regardless of your physical capabilities or medical diagnoses.

Here are the best ways to lose weight after 50.

LEARN TO ENJOY STRENGTH TRAINING

Although cardio gets a lot of attention when it comes to weight loss, strength training is also important, especially for older adults.

As you age, your muscle mass declines in a process called sarcopenia. This loss of muscle mass begins around the age of 50 and can slow your metabolism, which may lead to weight gain.

After the age of 50, your muscle mass decreases by about 1–2% per year, while your muscle strength declines at a rate of 1.5–5% per year.

Thus, adding muscle-building exercises to your routine is essential for reducing age-related muscle loss and promoting a healthy body weight.

Strength training, such as bodyweight exercises and weightlifting, can significantly improve muscle strength and increase muscle size and function.

Plus, strength training can help you lose weight by reducing body fat and boosting your metabolism, which can increase how many calories you burn throughout the day.

TEAM UP

Introducing a healthy eating pattern or exercise routine on your own can be challenging. Pairing up with a friend, co-worker, or family member may give you a better chance at sticking to your plan and achieving your wellness goals. For example, research shows that those who attend weight loss programs with friends are significantly more likely to maintain their weight loss over time.

Additionally, working out with friends can strengthen your commitment to a fitness program and make exercising more enjoyable.

SIT LESS AND MOVE MORE

Burning more calories than you take in is critical to losing excess body fat. That's why being more active throughout the day is important when trying to lose weight.

For example, sitting at your job for long periods of time might impede your weight loss efforts. To counteract this, you can become more active at work by simply getting up from your desk and taking a five-minute walk every hour.

Research shows that tracking your steps using a pedometer or Fitbit can boost weight loss by increasing your activity levels and calorie expenditure.

When using a pedometer or Fitbit, start with a realistic step goal based on your current activity levels. Then gradually work your way up to 7,000–10,000 steps per day or more, depending on your overall health.

BUMP UP YOUR PROTEIN INTAKE

Getting enough high-quality protein in your diet is not only important for weight loss but also critical for stopping or reversing age-related muscle loss.

How many calories you burn at rest, or your resting metabolic rate (RMR), decreases by 1–2% each decade after you turn 20. This is associated with age-related muscle loss.

However, eating a protein-rich diet can help prevent or even reverse muscle loss. Numerous studies have also shown that increasing dietary protein can help you lose weight and keep it off in the long.

Plus, research shows that older adults have higher protein needs than younger adults, making it all the more important to add protein-rich foods to your meals and snacks.

TALK TO A DIETITIAN

Finding an eating pattern that both promotes weight loss and nourishes your body can be difficult.

Consulting a registered dietitian can help you determine the best way to lose excess body fat without having to follow an overly restrictive diet. In addition, a dietitian can support and guide you throughout your weight loss journey.

Research shows that working with a dietitian to lose weight can lead to significantly better results than going at it alone, and it may help you maintain the weight loss over time.

COOK MORE AT HOME

Numerous studies have demonstrated that people who prepare and eat more meals at home tend to follow a healthier diet and weigh less than those who don't.

Cooking meals at home allows you to control what goes in — and what stays out — of your recipes. It also lets you experiment with unique, healthy ingredients that pique your interest.

If you eat most meals out of the house, start by cooking one or two meals per week at home, then gradually increase this number until you're cooking at home more than you eat out.

EAT MORE PRODUCE

Vegetables and fruits are packed with nutrients that are vital to your health, and adding them into your diet is a simple, evidence-based way to drop excess weight.

For example, a review of 10 studies found that every daily serving increase of vegetables was associated with a 0.14-inch (0.36-cm) waist circumference reduction in women.

Another study in 26,340 men and women aged 35–65 associated eating fruits and vegetables with lower body weight, reduced waist circumference, and less body fat.

HIRE A PERSONAL TRAINER

Working with a personal trainer can especially benefit those who are new to working out by teaching you the correct way to exercise to promote weight loss and avoiding injury.

Plus, personal trainers can motivate you to work out more by keeping you accountable. They may even improve your attitude about exercising.

A 10-week study in 129 adults showed that one-on-one personal training for 1 hour per week increased motivation to exercise and increased physical activity levels.

RELY LESS ON CONVENIENCE FOODS

Regularly eating convenience foods, such as fast food, candy, and processed snacks, is associated with weight gain and may hinder your weight loss efforts.

Convenience foods are typically high in calories and tend to be low in important nutrients like protein, fiber, vitamins, and minerals. That's why fast food and other processed foods are commonly referred to as "empty calories."

Cutting back on convenience foods and replacing them with nutritious meals and snacks that revolve around nutrient-dense whole foods is a smart way to lose weight.

FIND AN ACTIVITY THAT YOU LOVE

Finding an exercise routine that you can maintain long term can be difficult. This is why it's important to engage in activities that you enjoy.

For example, if you like group activities, sign up for a group sport like soccer or a running club so you can exercise with others on a regular basis.

If solo activities are more your style, try biking, walking, hiking, or swimming on your own.

GET CHECKED BY A HEALTHCARE PROVIDER

If you are struggling to lose weight even though you're active and follow a healthy diet, ruling out conditions that may make it difficult to lose weight — like hypothyroidism and polycystic ovarian syndrome (PCOS) — may be warranted.

This may be especially true if you have family members with these conditions.

Tell your healthcare provider about your symptoms so they can decide the best testing protocol to rule out medical conditions that may be behind your weight loss struggles.

EAT A WHOLE-FOODS-BASED DIET

One of the simplest ways to ensure that you give your body the nutrients it needs to thrive is by following a diet rich in whole foods.

Whole foods, including vegetables, fruits, nuts, seeds, poultry, fish, legumes, and grains, are packed with nutrients essential for maintaining a healthy body weight, such as fiber, protein, and healthy fats.

In many studies, whole-food-based diets, both plant-based diets and those that include animal products, have been associated with weight loss.

EAT LESS AT NIGHT

Many studies have shown that eating fewer calories at night may help you maintain a healthy body weight and lose excess body fat.

A study in 1,245 people found that over 6 years, those who consumed more calories at dinner were over 2 times more likely to become obese than people who ate more calories earlier in the day.

Plus, those who ate more calories at dinner were significantly more likely to develop metabolic syndrome, a group of conditions including high blood sugar and excess belly fat. Metabolic syndrome increases your risk of heart disease, diabetes, and stroke.

Eating the majority of your calories during breakfast and lunch, while enjoying a lighter dinner, may be a worthwhile method to promote weight loss.

FOCUS ON BODY COMPOSITION

Although body weight is a good indicator of health, your body composition — meaning the percentages of fat and fat-free mass in your body — is important as well.

Muscle mass is an important measure of overall health, especially in older adults.

Packing on more muscle and losing excess fat should be your goal.

There are many ways to measure your body fat percentage. However, simply measuring your waist, biceps, calves, chest, and thighs can help you determine if you're losing fat and gaining muscle.

HYDRATE THE HEALTHY WAY

Drinks like sweetened coffee beverages, soda, juices, sports drinks, and pre-made smoothies are often packed with calories and added sugars.

Drinking sugar-sweetened beverages, especially those sweetened with high-fructose corn syrup, is strongly linked to weight gain and conditions like obesity, heart disease, diabetes, and fatty liver disease.

Swapping sugary beverages with healthy drinks like water and herbal tea can help you lose weight and may significantly reduce your risk of developing the chronic conditions mentioned above.

CHOOSE THE RIGHT SUPPLEMENTS

If you feel fatigued and unmotivated, taking the right supplements may help give you the energy you need to reach your goals.

As you grow older, your ability to absorb certain nutrients declines, increasing your risk of deficiencies. For example, research shows that adults over 50 are commonly deficient in folate and vitamin B12, two nutrients that are needed for energy production.

Deficiencies in B vitamins like B12 can negatively impact your mood, cause fatigue, and hinder weight loss.

For this reason, it's a good idea for those over 50 to take a high-quality B-complex vitamin to help decrease the risk of deficiency.

LIMIT ADDED SUGARS

Limiting foods high in added sugar, including sweetened beverages, candy, cakes, cookies, ice cream, sweetened yogurts, and sugary cereals, is critical for weight loss at any age.

Because sugar is added to so many foods, including items that you wouldn't expect like tomato sauce, salad dressing, and bread, reading ingredient labels is the best way to determine if an item contains added sugar.

Look for "added sugars" on the nutrition facts label or search the ingredient list for common sweeteners such as cane sugar, high-fructose corn syrup, and agave.

IMPROVE YOUR SLEEP QUALITY

Not getting enough quality sleep may harm your weight loss efforts. Many studies have shown that not getting enough sleep increases the likelihood of obesity and may hinder weight loss efforts.

For example, a 2-year study in 245 women demonstrated that those who slept 7 hours per night or more were 33% more likely to lose weight than women who slept less than 7 hours per night. Better sleep quality was also associated with weight loss success.

Aim to get the recommended 7–9 hours of sleep per night and improve your sleep quality by minimizing light in your bedroom and avoiding using your phone or watching TV before bed.

TRY OUT INTERMITTENT FASTING

Intermittent fasting is a type of eating pattern in which you only eat during a specified period. The most popular type of intermittent fasting is the 16/8 method, where you eat within an 8-hour window followed by a 16-hour fast.

Numerous studies have shown that intermittent fasting promotes weight loss.

What's more, some test-tube and animal studies suggest that intermittent fasting may benefit older adults by increasing longevity, slowing cell decline, and preventing age-related changes to mitochondria, the energy-producing parts of your cells.

BE MORE MINDFUL

Mindful eating can be a simple way to improve your relationship with food, all while encouraging weight loss.

Mindful eating involves paying more attention to your food and eating patterns. It gives you a better understanding of your hunger and fullness cues, as well as how food impacts your mood and well-being.

Many studies have noted that using mindful eating techni？ues promotes weight loss and improves eating behaviors.

There are no specific rules to mindful eating, but eating slowly, paying attention to the aroma and flavor of each bite of food, and keeping track of how you feel during your meals are simple ways to introduce mindful eating to your life.

The Bottom Line…

Though weight loss may seem to get more difficult with age, many evidence-based strategies can help you achieve and maintain a healthy body weight after turning 50.

Cutting out added sugars, incorporating strength training into your workouts, eating more protein, cooking meals at home, and following a whole-foods-based diet are just some of the methods you can use to improve your overall health and lose excess body fat.

Try out the tips above, and before you know it, weight loss after 50 will seem like a breeze.

COMMON MISTAKES

1. STARTING OFF DRASTICALLY WITH INTERMITTENT FASTING

Starting off drastically is one of the biggest mistakes you can make. If you jump into IF without easing into it, you may set yourself up for disaster. Going from eating 3 normal sized meals or 6 small meals per day to eating within a four-hour window, for example, can be a tough adjustment.

Instead, ease into fasting gradually. If you are aiming for the 16/8 method, slowly extend the times between meals until you can comfortably work within a 12-hour window. Then, to reduce the window to 8 hours, add several minutes per day until you get to the 8-hour window.

2. NOT CHOOSING THE RIGHT PLAN FOR INTERMITTENT FASTING

You're ready to try Intermittent Fasting for weight loss and have grocery shopped for whole foods like fish and chicken, fruits and veggies, and healthy sides like quinoa and legumes. The problem is, you haven't chosen the IF plan that will set you up for success. If you are a dedicated gym-goer 6 days a week, completely fasting for two of those days may not be the ideal plan.

Rather than jump into a plan without thinking, analyze your lifestyle a little and consider the plan than will fit your schedule and habits best.

3. EATING TOO MUCH IN YOUR FASTING WINDOW

One of the reasons people choose to try Intermittent Fasting is that the reduced time available to eat means consuming fewer calories. However, some people will eat their usual number of calories in the span of the fasting window. This may mean that you will not lose weight.

Don't eat your regular consumption of say, 2000 calories in the window. Instead, plan to eat around 1200 to 1500 calories during the period when you break the fast. How many meals you eat will depend on the length of the fasting window, whether it be 4, 6, or 8 hours. If you need to overeat and are in a state of deprivation, reconsider the plan you chose to follow, or ease off the IF for a day to refocus and then get back on track.

4. EATING THE WRONG FOODS IN YOUR FASTING WINDOW

The Intermittent Fasting mistake of eating the wrong foods runs hand in hand with overeating. If you have a fasting window of 6 hours and fill it with refined, fatty, or sugary foods, you are not going to feel well at all.

Lean proteins, healthy fats, nuts, legumes, unrefined grains, and wholesome veggies and fruits become the mainstay of your diet. As well, in between fasting, follow these clean eating tips:

• Cook and eat at home as opposed to in a restaurant

• Read nutrition labels and become familiar with forbidden ingredients like high fructose corn syrup and modified palm oil

• Watch your sodium intake and beware of hidden sugars

• Avoid processed foods and cook whole foods instead

• Balance your plate with fiber, healthy carbs and fats, and lean proteins

5. RESTRICTING CALORIES IN YOUR FASTING WINDOW

Yes, there is such a thing as reducing your calories too much. Eating less than 1200 calories in your fasting window is not healthy. Not only that, but it can also sabotage your metabolic rate. If you slow your metabolism down too much, you will begin to lose muscle mass as opposed to increasing it.

To avoid this mistake, try prepping your food for the week ahead on the weekend. This gives you balanced, healthy meals ready at your fingertips. When it is time to eat, you can enjoy a healthy, nutritious, and caloric-correct meal.

6. UNKNOWINGLY BREAKING THE INTERMITTENT FAST

Hidden fast breakers are something you should be aware of. Did you know that even the taste of sweetness triggers your brain's insulin response? This causes an insulin release and can effectively break the fast. Here is a look at surprise foods, supplements, and products that can bring a fast to a halt and cause an insulin response:

• Supplements that contain additives like maltodextrin and pectin

• Vitamins, such as gummy bear vitamins, contain sugar and fat

• Using toothpaste and mouthwash containing the sweetener xylitol

• Pain relievers such as Advil can have sugar in the coating

Don't make the Intermittent Fasting mistake of breaking your fast. Use a baking soda and water paste to brush your teeth when in a non-eating period and read the labels carefully before taking vitamins and supplements.

7. NOT DRINKING ENOUGH WHEN INTERMITTENT FASTING

Staying hydrated is an important part of IF. Remember, your body is not taking in the water that would be consumed with food. Because of this, side effects can derail you if you are not careful. Headaches, muscle cramps, and intense feelings of hunger can quickly appear if you allow yourself to become dehydrated.

To avoid this mistake and ward off annoying symptoms like cramping and headaches, include the following in your day:

• Water

• Water and 1-2 tbsp of apple cider vinegar (this may even curb your hunger)

- Black coffee

- Black, herbal, oolong, or green tea

8. NOT EXERCISING WHEN INTERMITTENT FASTING

Some people think they can't exercise when in a period of IF, when in fact, it's the ideal scenario. Exercise helps you use up stored fat. Additionally, the Human Growth Hormone is increased as you work out, helping you to build muscle. However, there are tips to follow to maximize your workouts.

To get the best results from your efforts, keep these points in mind:

• Time your workouts for during the eating periods and then eat healthy carbs and proteins within 30 minutes of the exercise

• If the type of exercise is intense, make sure you eat before so that your glycogen stores are available

• Base your exercise on the fasting method; if you are doing a 24 hour fast, do not plan an intensive activity that day

• Stay hydrated during the fast and especially during the workout

• Listen to your body's signals; if you feel weak or light-headed, take a break or conclude the workout

9. BEING TOO HARD ON YOURSELF IF YOU SLIP WHEN INTERMITTENT FASTING

One slip does not a failure make! Sometimes you'll have days when an IF regimen is extra tough, and you just don't think you can make it. It's totally okay to take a break if you need to. Give yourself a day to refocus. Stay on a healthy eating track but allow yourself treats like an awesome protein smoothie or a serving of healthy beef and broccoli and jump back in the next day.

Don't make the mistake of allowing Intermittent Fasting to consume your whole life. Consider a part of your healthy lifestyle and remember to do other important things for yourself, too. Enjoy a book, exercise, spend time with the family, and eat as healthily as you can. It's all part of the package of being the best you can be.

10. USING IT AS AN EXCUSE TO EAT RUBBISH

Unfortunately, people think that intermittent fasting is a magic pill that will solve all their problems. Yes, it is an incredibly effective tool to take control of your health but it won't cancel out eating a diet full of processed foods and sugar. When you are intermittent fasting it is even more important to nourish your body with nutrient dense, whole foods.

When you are in the fasted state, your body starts to break down damaged components and then uses them for of energy, this process cleans and heals the body. It also means your body becomes more sensitive to the food you eat, this is great if it's full of nutrients to nourish the body, but not good if you are eating rubbish.

Not only that, if you aren't nourishing yourself with nutrient dense foods, you will feel hungry all the time – your body will crave nutrients.

11. TRYING TO CALORIE RESTRICT DURING THE 'EATING WINDOW'

One of the main issues that some people face when they start IF is that they continue to calorie restrict when they have broken their fast. The whole point of eating in this way is to listen to your body and start eating until you feel full.

Your body is an amazing machine, if you allow it to do its job properly. Your body will release hormones to make you feel full when it knows it's had enough food. If you calorie restrict during your eating window you may well end up under eating which causes lots of unwanted changes in the body, and long term is not good for you.

12. ATTEMPTING TO DO TOO MANY THINGS AT ONCE – OVER TRAIN, UNDER EAT AND TRY FASTING

If you have spent a number of years eating badly and not exercising and you would like to try IF, don't bite off more than you can chew (pun intended!) at the start. Ease yourself into fasting and training gradually; don't start training five times per week, fasting every day and restricting calories when you do eat from day one.

The combination can lead to problems. Your body thrives with a little bit of physical stress here and there but too much stress can create chronic issues.

13. OBSESSING OVER TIMINGS AND 'EATING WINDOWS'

In my opinion, one of the main benefits of IF is teaching you to become completely in tune with your body and understand what I call 'real hunger' – something that occurs every 16-24 hours, not every four hours.

Your body should dictate when you should eat, not the clock. If you focus on time periods, you end up counting down the hours until you can eat – you never learn to understand your bodies signals.

14. NOT DRINKING ENOUGH WATER

When your body is in the fasted state it starts to break down damaged components and detoxifies the body. It is very important that you flush out those toxins by drinking lots of water. Ideally, you will drink more water than you usually would. I drink roughly four-fiver liters every day, most of that during my fasting period.

Not only that, drinking water, particularly sparkling water can help you to feel full, which is important when you are first getting into IF.

INTERMITTENT FASTING RECIPES

1. Egg Scramble with Sweet Potatoes

Total time: 25 minutes | Servings: 1

Ingredients:

- 1 (8-oz) sweet potato, diced

- ½ cup chopped onion

- 2 tsp chopped rosemary

- Salt

- Pepper

- 4 large eggs

- 4 large egg whites

- 2 tbsp chopped chive

Directions:

1. Preheat the oven to 425°F. On a baking sheet, toss the sweet potato, onion, rosemary, and salt and pepper. Spray with cooking spray and roast until tender, about 20 minutes.

2. Meanwhile, in a medium bowl, whisk together the eggs, egg whites, and a pinch of salt and pepper. Spritz a skillet with cooking spray and scramble the eggs on medium, about 5 minutes.

3. Sprinkle with chopped chives and serve with the spuds.

Per serving: 571 calories, 44 g protein, 52 g carbs (9 g fiber), 20 g fat

2. Greek Chickpea Waffles

Total time: 30 minutes | Servings: 2

Ingredients:

- ¾ cup chickpea flour

- ½ tsp baking soda

- ½ tsp salt

- ¾ cup plain 2% Greek yogurt

- 6 large eggs

• Tomatoes, cucumbers, scallion, olive oil, parsley, yogurt, and lemon juice for serving (optional)

• Salt and pepper

Directions:

1. Preheat the oven to 200°F. Set a wire rack over a rimmed baking sheet and place in the oven. Heat a waffle iron per directions.

2. In a large bowl, whisk together the flour, baking soda, and salt. In a small bowl, whisk together the yogurt and eggs. Stir the wet ingredients into the dry ingredients.

3. Lightly coat the waffle iron with nonstick cooking spray. In batches, drop ¼ to ½ cup batter into each section of the iron and cook until golden brown, 4 to 5 minutes. Transfer the waffles to the oven and keep warm. Repeat with remaining batter.

4. Serve waffles with the savory tomato mix or a drizzle of warm nut butter and berries.

Per serving: 412 calories, 35 g protein, 24 g carbs (4 g fiber), 18 g fat

3. PB&J Overnight Oats

Total time: 5 minutes (plus 8 hours for refrigeration) | Servings: 1

Ingredients:

- ¼ cup quick-cooking rolled oats
- ½ cup 2 percent milk
- 3 tbsp creamy peanut butter
- ¼ cup mashed raspberries
- 3 tbsp whole raspberries

Directions:

1. In a medium bowl, combine oats, milk, peanut butter, and mashed raspberries. Stir until smooth.

2. Cover and refrigerate overnight. In the morning, uncover and top with whole raspberries.

Per serving: 455 calories, 20 g protein, 36 g carbs (9 g fiber), 28 g fat

4. Turmeric Tofu Scramble

Total time: 15 minutes | Servings: 1

Ingredients:

- 1 portobello mushroom

- 3 or 4 cherry tomatoes

- 1 tbsp olive oil, plus more for brushing

- Salt and pepper

- ½ block (14-oz) firm tofu

- ¼ tsp ground turmeric

- Pinch garlic powder

- ½ avocado, thinly sliced

Directions:

1. Preheat the oven to 400°F. On a baking sheet, place the shroom and

tomatoes and brush them with oil. Season with salt and pepper. Roast until tender, about 10 minutes.

2. Meanwhile, in a medium bowl, combine the tofu, turmeric, garlic powder, and a pinch of salt. Mash with a fork. In a large skillet over medium, heat 1 Tbsp olive oil. Add the tofu mixture and cook, stirring occasionally, until firm and egg-like, about 3 minutes.

3. Plate the tofu and serve with the mushroom, tomatoes, and avocado.

Per serving: 431 calories, 21 g protein, 17 g carbs (8 g fiber), 33 g fat

5. Avocado Ricotta Power Toast

Total time: 5 minutes | Servings: 1

Ingredients:

- 1 slice whole-grain bread

- ¼ ripe avocado, smashed

- 2 tbsp ricotta

- Pinch crushed red pepper flakes
- Pinch flaky sea salt

Directions:

1. Toast the bread. Top with avocado, ricotta, crushed red pepper flakes, and sea salt. Eat with scrambled or hard-boiled eggs, plus a serving of yogurt or fruit.

Per serving: 288 calories, 10 g protein, 29 g carbs (10 g fiber), 17 g fat

6. Turkish Egg Breakfast

Total time: 13 minutes | Servings: 2

Ingredients:

- 2 tbsp olive oil
- ¾ cup diced red bell pepper
- ¾ cup diced eggplant
- Pinch each of salt and pepper

- 5 large eggs, lightly beaten

- ¼ tsp paprika

- Chopped cilantro, to taste

- 2 dollops plain yogurt

- 1 whole-wheat pita

Directions:

1. In a large nonstick skillet on medium high, heat the olive oil. Add the bell pepper, eggplant, and salt and pepper. Sauté until softened, about 7 minutes.

2. Stir in the eggs, paprika, and more salt and pepper to taste. Cook, stirring often, until the eggs are softly scrambled.

3. Sprinkle with chopped cilantro and serve with a dollop of yogurt and the pita.

Per serving: 469 calories, 25 g protein, 26 g carbs (4 g fiber), 29 g fat

7. Almond Apple Spice Muffins

Total time: 15 minutes | Servings: 5

Ingredients:

- ½ stick butter
- 2 cups almond meal
- 4 scoops vanilla protein powder
- 4 large eggs
- 1 cup unsweetened applesauce
- 1 tbsp cinnamon
- 1 tsp allspice
- 1 tsp cloves
- 2 tsp baking powder

Directions:

1. Preheat the oven to 350°F. In a small microwave-safe bowl, melt the butter in the microwave on low heat, about 30 seconds.

2. In a large bowl, thoroughly mix all the remaining ingredients with the melted butter. Spray 2 muffin tins with nonstick cooking spray or use cupcake liners.

3. Pour the mixture into the muffin tins, making sure not to overfill (about ¾ full). This should make 10 muffins.

4. Place one tray in the oven and bake for 12 minutes. Make sure not to overbake, as the muffins will become too dry. When baked, remove the first tray from the oven and bake the second muffin tin the same way.

Per serving: 484 calories, 40 g protein, 16 g carbs (5 g fiber), 31 g fat

DINNER RECIPES

1. Turkey Tacos

Total time: 25 minutes | Servings: 4

Ingredients:

- 2 tsp oil

- 1 small red onion, chopped

- 1 clove garlic, finely chopped

- 1 lb. extra-lean ground turkey

- 1 tbsp sodium-free taco seasoning

- 8 whole-grain corn tortillas, warmed

- ¼ cup sour cream

- ½ cup shredded Mexican cheese

- 1 avocado, sliced

- Salsa, for serving

- 1 cup chopped lettuce

Directions:

1. In a large skillet on medium high, heat the oil. Add the onion and cook, stirring until tender, 5 to 6 minutes. Stir in the garlic and cook 1 minute.

2. Add the turkey and cook, breaking it up with a spoon, until nearly brown, 5

minutes. Add the taco seasoning and 1 cup water. Simmer until reduced by slightly more than half, 7 minutes.

3. Fill the tortillas with turkey and top with sour cream, cheese, avocado, salsa, and lettuce.

Per serving: 472 calories, 28 g protein, 30 g carbs (6 g fiber), 27 g fat

2. Healthy Spaghetti Bolognese

Total time: 1 hour 30 minutes | Servings: 4

Ingredients:

- 1 large spaghetti squash

- 3 tbsp olive oil

- ½ tsp garlic powder

- Kosher salt and pepper

- 1 small onion, finely chopped

- 1¼ lb. ground turkey

- 4 cloves garlic, finely chopped

- 8 oz. small cremini mushrooms, sliced

- 3 cups fresh diced tomatoes (or 2 15-oz cans)

- 1 (8-oz) can low-sodium, no-sugar-added tomato sauce

- Fresh chopped basil

Directions:

1. Preheat the oven to 400°F. Cut the spaghetti squash in half lengthwise and discard seeds. Rub each half with 1/2 tbsp oil and season with garlic powder and ¼ tsp each salt and pepper. Place skin-side up on a rimmed baking sheet and roast until tender, 35 to 40 minutes. Let cool for 10 minutes.

2. Meanwhile, in a large skillet on medium, heat remaining 2 Tbsp oil. Add the onion, season with ¼ tsp each salt and pepper, and cook, stirring occasionally, until tender, 6 minutes. Add the turkey and cook, breaking it up into small pieces with a spoon, until

browned, 6 to 7 minutes. Stir in the garlic and cook 1 minute.

3. Push the turkey mixture to one side of the pan, and add the mushrooms to the other. Cook, stirring occasionally, until the mushrooms are tender, 5 minutes. Mix into the turkey. Add the tomatoes and tomato sauce and simmer for 10 minutes.

4. While the sauce is simmering, scoop out the squash and transfer to plates. Spoon the turkey Bolognese over the top and sprinkle with basil, if desired.

Per serving: 450 calories, 32 g protein, 31 g carbs (6 g fiber), 23 g fat

3. Chicken with Fried Cauliflower Rice

Total time: 35 minutes | Servings: 4

Ingredients:

• 2 tbsp grapeseed oil

• 1 ¼ lb. boneless, skinless chicken breast, pounded to even thickness

- 4 large eggs, beaten

- 2 red bell peppers, finely chopped

- 2 small carrots, finely chopped

- 1 onion, finely chopped

- 2 cloves garlic, finely chopped

- 4 scallions, finely chopped, plus more for serving

- ½ cup frozen peas, thawed

- 4 cups cauliflower "rice"

- 2 tbsp low-sodium soy sauce

- 2 tsp rice vinegar

- Kosher salt and pepper

Directions:

1. In a large, deep skillet over medium-high, heat 1 tbsp oil. Add the chicken and cook until golden brown, 3 to 4 minutes per side. Transfer to a cutting board and let rest for 6 minutes before slicing. Add remaining 1 tbsp oil to the

skillet. Add the eggs and scramble until just set, 1 to 2 minutes; transfer to a bowl.

2. To the skillet, add the bell pepper, carrot, and onion and cook, stirring often until just tender, 4 to 5 minutes. Stir in the garlic and cook, 1 minute. Toss with scallions and peas.

3. Add the cauliflower, soy sauce, rice vinegar, salt and pepper and toss to combine. Then let the cauliflower sit, without stirring, until beginning to brown, 2 to 3 minutes. Toss with the sliced chicken and eggs.

Per serving: 427 calories, 45 g protein, 25 g carbs (7 g fiber), 16 g fat

4. Sheet Pan Steak

Total time: 50 minutes | Servings: 4

Ingredients:

• 1 lb. small cremini mushrooms, trimmed and halved

- 1 ¼ lb. bunch broccolini, trimmed and cut into 2-in. lengths

- 4 cloves garlic, finely chopped

- 3 tbsp olive oil

- ¼ tsp red pepper flakes (or a bit more for extra kick)

- Kosher salt and pepper

- 2 1-in.-thick New York strip steaks (about 1½ lb total), trimmed of excess fat

- 1 15-oz can low-sodium cannellini beans, rinsed

Directions:

1. Preheat the oven to 450°F. On a large rimmed baking sheet, toss the mushrooms, broccolini, garlic, oil, red pepper flakes, and ¼ tsp each salt and pepper. Place the baking sheet in the oven and roast 15 minutes.

2. Push the mixture to the edges of the pan to make room for the steaks. Season

the steaks with ¼ tsp each salt and pepper and place in the center of the pan. Roast the steaks to desired doneness, 5 to 7 minutes per side for medium-rare. Transfer the steaks to a cutting board and let rest 5 minutes before slicing.

3. Add the beans to the baking sheet and toss to combine. Roast until heated through, about 3 minutes. Serve beans and vegetables with steak.

Per serving: 464 calories, 42 g protein, 26 g carbs (8 g fiber), 22 g fat

5. Pork Tenderloin with Butternut Squash and Brussels Sprouts

Total time: 50 minutes | Servings: 4

Ingredients:

- 1 ¾ lb. pork tenderloin, trimmed

- Salt

- Pepper

- 3 tbsp canola oil

- 2 sprigs fresh thyme

- 2 garlic cloves, peeled

- 4 cups Brussels sprouts, trimmed and halved

- 4 cups diced butternut squash

Directions:

1. Preheat the oven to 400°F. Season the tenderloin all over with salt and pepper. In a large cast-iron pan over medium high, heat 1 tbsp oil. When the oil shimmers, add the tenderloin and sear until golden brown on all sides, 8 to 12 minutes total. Transfer to a plate.

2. Add the thyme and garlic and remaining 2 tbsp oil to the pan and cook until aromatic, about 1 minute. Add the Brussels sprouts, the butternut squash, and a big pinch each of salt and pepper. Cook, stirring occasionally, until the vegetables are slightly browned, 4 to 6 minutes.

3. Place the tenderloin atop the vegetables and transfer everything to the oven. Roast until the vegetables are tender and a meat thermometer inserted into the thickest part of the tenderloin registers 140°F, 15 to 20 minutes.

4. Wearing oven mitts, carefully remove the pan from the oven. Allow the tenderloin to rest 5 minutes before slicing and serving with the vegetables. Toss greens with a balsamic vinaigrette to serve as a side.

Per serving: 401 calories, 44 g protein, 25 g carbs (6 g fiber), 15 g fat

6. Wild Cajun Spiced Salmon

Total time: 30 minutes | Servings: 4

Ingredients:

- 1½ lb. wild Alaskan salmon fillet

- Sodium-free taco seasoning

- ½ head cauliflower (about 1 lb), cut into florets

- 1 head broccoli (about 1 lb), cut into florets

- 3 tbsp olive oil

- ½ tsp garlic powder

- 4 medium tomatoes, diced

Directions:

1. Preheat the oven to 375°F. Place the salmon in a baking dish. In a small bowl, mix the taco seasoning with ½ cup water. Pour the mixture over the salmon and bake until opaque throughout, 12 to 15 minutes.

2. Meanwhile, in a food processor (in batches as necessary), pulse the cauliflower and broccoli until finely chopped and "riced."

3. In a large skillet on medium, heat the oil. Add the cauliflower and broccoli, sprinkle with garlic powder, and cook, tossing until just tender, 5 to 6 minutes.

4. Serve salmon on top of "rice" and top with tomatoes.

Per serving: 408 calories, 42 g protein, 9 g carbs (3 g fiber), 23 g fat

7. Pork Chops with Bloody Mary Tomato Salad

Total time: 25 minutes | Servings: 4

Ingredients:

- 2 tbsp olive oil

- 2 tbsp red wine vinegar

- 2 tsp Worcestershire sauce

- 2 tsp prepared horseradish, squeezed dry

- ½ tsp Tabasco

- ½ tsp celery seeds

- Kosher salt

- 1 pint cherry tomatoes, halved

- 2 celery stalks, very thinly sliced

- ½ small red onion, thinly sliced

- 4 small bone-in pork chops (1 in. thick, about 2¼ lb total)

- Pepper

- ¼ cup finely chopped flat-leaf parsley

- 1 small head green-leaf lettuce, leaves torn

Directions:

1. Heat grill to medium high. In a large bowl, whisk together the oil, vinegar, Worcestershire sauce, horseradish, Tabasco, celery seeds, and ¼ tsp salt. Toss with the tomatoes, celery, and onion.

2. Season the pork chops with ½ tsp each salt and pepper and grill until golden brown and just cooked through, 5 to 7 minutes per side.

3. Fold the parsley into the tomatoes and serve over pork and greens. Eat with mashed cauliflower or potatoes.

Per serving: 400 calories, 39 g protein, 8 g carbs (3 g fiber), 23 g fat

Manufactured by Amazon.ca
Bolton, ON